IMPORTANT NOTICE FOR THOSE WHO WISH TO ENROLL IN THE CORRESPONDENCE COURSE.

If you wish to take *Homeopathic Medicine in the Home* as a correspondence course and receive individualized guidance, tutoring, and evaluation, with a certificate of achievement upon completion of the course: Fill out the attached **Order Form - Enrollment/Disclaimer Statement** and remit it with payment of $230.00 to:

ASHWINS PUBLICATIONS
POST OFFICE BOX 1686
OJAI, CALIFORNIA 93024

D1591983

FOREIGN STUDENTS: Please add $15.00 to cover air mail correspondence. All foreign enrollments must be paid in U.S. dollars drawn on a U.S. bank. Canadian students add $7.00 to U.S. rates.

NOTE: The $230.00 Enrollment Fee entitles you to a maximum of 14 months of course tutoring. As is explained on p. 2 of this Course Syllabus, the course may be completed at the rate of one lesson per week, or in 3 months. The average completion time is between 3-8 months. There will be an extra fee of $35.00 for every 2 lessons of written assignments if they are sent in after 14 months from the date of receipt of the Enrollment/ Disclaimer Statement by Ashwins Publications. The maximum course completion time is 3 years.

REQUIRED COURSE TEXTS
You must also have these 2 supplementary texts in order to begin the course. These texts are listed on p. 1 of this Course Syllabus, they are:

Homeopathic Medicine at Home, by Panos and Heimlich
Materia Medica with Repertory, by Boericke

These supplementary texts may be obtained from the same source where you bought this Course Syllabus. If you have difficulty finding these books, they are obtainable from Ashwins Publications or from the sources listed on p. 134 of this Course Syllabus.

You can take *Homeopathic Medicine in the Home* as a correspondence course with individualized tutoring *ONLY* when the tutoring fee of $230.00 is paid and the **Order-Form Enrollment/Disclaimer Statement** is completed and sent to Ashwins Publications. Prices subject to change.

ORDER FORM

Individualized Correspondence Tutoring
with Certificate of Achievement
upon Completion $230.00

PAYMENT BY: ☐ VISA ☐ M/C ☐ Check ☐ Money Order

Card No: ☐☐☐☐☐☐☐☐☐☐☐☐☐☐☐☐ Exp. Date ☐☐ (MO. YR.) _____
CARDHOLDER'S SIGNATURE

Foreign Students: Please add $15.00 to cover air mail correspondence. All foreign enrollments must be paid in U.S. dollars drawn on a U.S. bank.
Canadian students add $7.00 to U.S. rates.
Prices subject to change

Make checks payable to: ASHWINS PUBLICATIONS
Mail Order Form with payment to:
ASHWINS PUBLICATIONS
Post Office Box 1686
Ojai, California 93024
(805) 646-6622

NOTE: You must have the 2 supplementary texts, *Homeopathic Medicine at Home* by Panos and Heimlich, and *Materia Medica with Repertory* by Boericke, in order to begin the course. If you have difficulty in obtaining these texts, they may be ordered by contacting Ashwins Publications at the address and phone given on this card.

ENROLLMENT/DISCLAIMER STATEMENT

Complete this card and send it in to Ashwins Publications ONLY if you are enrolling in the correspondence course with individualized tutoring and paying the course tutor fee.

Homeopathic Medicine in the Home is solely intended to provide a format to assist the student in learning and applying the principles of homeopathy. However, the material contained in this course is in no way to be considered as a substitute for consultation with a licensed health professional. This course book is a reference work and is not intended to provide diagnosis, prescription or treatment. Ashwins Publications and the author cannot make any claims concerning the benefits of homeopathy in individual medical situations. In addition, although homeopathy is safe and gentle when used in accordance with the guidelines given in the course, Ashwins Publications and the author cannot assume liability for any effects resulting from the student's use of homeopathy. Therefore, all enrollees in the course must sign the following statement before they will be accepted in the course:

I hereby release Ashwins Publications and the author from any responsibility or liability resulting from my use of homeopathic medicines for myself and/or others. By enrolling in *Homeopathic Medicine in the Home* I assume sole responsibility for my use of homeopathic principles or medicines. I understand that the material contained in this course is not to be considered as a substitute for consultation with a licensed health professional.

NAME (Please Print)   SIGNATURE   DATE

ADDRESS — STREET   CITY   STATE/COUNTRY   ZIP

TELEPHONE   OCCUPATION   AGE

HOMEOPATHIC
MEDICINE
IN THE HOME

a correspondence study course

HOMEOPATHIC MEDICINE
IN THE HOME
a correspondence study course

by
Jonathan Breslow

foreword by
Karl Robinson, M.D.

ASHWINS PUBLICATIONS • OJAI • CALIFORNIA

DISCLAIMER
Homeopathic Medicine in the Home is solely intended to provide a format to assist the student in learning and applying the principles of homeopathy. However, the material contained in this course is in no way to be considered as a substitute for consultation with a licensed health professional. This course book is a reference work and is not intended to provide diagnosis, prescription or treatment.

ISBN 0-9620939-0-4

Library of Congress Catalog Card No.: 88-71470

Text Design by Heather Burney
Text Illustrations by Heather Burney and Kathy Hardin

Printed in the United States of America
First Edition 1988
2nd Printing 1990

Ashwins Publications
Post Office Box 1686
Ojai, California 93024

ACKNOWLEDGEMENTS

The concept of this course was initiated out of the vision and selfless support of Bonnie and Lawrence Williams of Oak Meadow School, innovators in the field of holistic education, to whom the author gives deepest thanks.

To those gifted individuals and organizations who have seen the vision and value of this course and offered assistance and support in its manifestation, I remain in gratitude. Those who most prominently come to mind are my parents, George and Florence Breslow, who have played an essential role in supporting the manifestation of this undertaking, also Santosh Krinsky of Lotus Light Publications, Dr. Maesimund B. Panos and Chakrapani Ullal. Special thanks to Bob and Heather Burney for their support and expertise in typography and graphic design and to David Farley for his editing work. Also thanks to the Happy Valley Foundation, the National Center for Homeopathy, the International Foundation for Homeopathy, Dr. A.S. Dalal, Jay Borneman, Marvin Banasky of the American Value Exchange, and to all others who have helped in this work.

The material offered in this course owes much of its origins to a galaxy of homeopathic physician-authors who have labored to provide a wealth of knowledge. To these past generations of homeopaths, as well as those contemporary teachers who have added to the author's knowledge, especially Robin Murphy, N.D., Dr. Francisco Eizayaga, and George Vithoulkas; appreciation and gratitude are offered.

A course of this nature which covers a broad area, bridging concepts and techniques, is bound to have its share of errors. These are the sole responsibility of the author.

DEDICATION

To George Breslow, S.A. and M.

FOREWORD

Homeopathy, I like to think, is Queen of Therapies. She can alleviate suffering and cure the sick more safely and thoroughly, yes, and often more quickly, than any other form of medicine. She performs her multifaceted miracles for the beginner as well as for the expert. After a mere five minutes of instruction *anyone* can learn to use *Arnica* and watch swollen injured tissue lose its swollen painfulness, if not in minutes, certainly in hours. There is perhaps no single medicine in our materia medica which so lends itself to the neophyte. To use *Arnica* is to prove to oneself and to the patient the efficacy of homeopathy. To see *Arnica* act compels one's attention. On the other hand, to cure endometriosis or rheumatoid arthritis might easily take even the determined practitioner years of careful study. But it has been done and it can be done. All that is needed is proper instruction and diligent application.

Although is is relatively easy to learn to use a few homeopathic remedies for first aid purposes - and that should definitely be one's first priority, one soon learns that treating common illnesses such as influenza, gut problems, and bed-wetting is not quite so easy. It is at this juncture, where one knows the remedies work and would like to be able to treat more comprehensively, that one begins to search for a book or course that will enable one's skills to grow.

Jonathan Breslow has created just such a course - *Homeopathic Medicine in the Home.* This correspondence study course is a well thought out series of lessons aimed at the beginning homeopath whether lay or professional. What is particularly reassuring about the course is that its sheet anchors are *Homeopathic Medicine at Home,* by Maesimund Panos, M.D., and *Materia Medica with Repertory,* by William Boericke, M.D., two basic works that all homeopaths can endorse.

Breslow has included important lessons on homeopathic philosophy, Hering's laws of cure, casetaking, and case analysis, as well as essential drilling on the common acute homeopathic remedies. The subscriber who takes the time to follow the lessons and work diligently should be well on the way to proficiency in homeopathic prescribing by the time the course has been completed.

As one proceeds through the lessons one begins to learn how to think like a homeopath. And thinking according to *similia similibus curentur* ("Let likes be cured by likes") is very different from the current medical model so popular in Western culture. Our culture is comfortable with the questions, "What medicines do you use to treat herpes?" or "What's the best peptic ulcer remedy?" but the homeopath *never* thinks that way. A homeopath always responds to such questions with, "It depends on the symptoms." He shows interest, albeit faint, in the condition to be treated yet becomes animated when his patient comes forth with a rare and unusual symptom. For the homeopath the credo is *individualization* . It is the unique individual patient before him that interests him far more than the diagnosis the patient carries. He doesn't treat diseases, per se, he treats the sick person before him.

This process of learning to think like a homeopath takes time and application but it is achievable and it is definitely worth doing. *Homeopathic Medicine in the Home* provides an excellent way of beginning this process.

Karl Robinson, M.D.
Albuquerque, N.M.

CONTENTS

List of Illustrations

INTRODUCTION

WELCOME TO
HOMEOPATHIC MEDICINE IN THE HOME!

Homeopathic Medicine in the Home is a correspondence study course which offers the knowledge and practical skills essential for resolving common ailments and injuries homeopathically. The course provides a lucid introduction to the art and science of homeopathy, while the techniques of case analysis are presented in a simple accessible format.

Homeopathy is a science and it is an art form. It is the subtle skills of homeopathy which make it an art form. Learning these skills is facilitated through the experience and guidance of an instructor. Throughout the course you will be receiving guidance and shared insights which come from experience. Your course instructor is here to help you, correct your Lesson Assignments, guide you in your learning and answer any questions which may arise.

The Lessons have been carefully designed to form a natural progression of learning stages which simplifies and demystifies an otherwise complex subject. We wish you an enjoyable and rewarding learning experience.

Note for anyone who is undergoing constitutional treatment[1] under the care of a homeopathic physician:
Before implementing homeopathic self-care on yourself it is essential to check with your practitioner to seek his or her approval. In some cases a homeopathic remedy, if taken on your own, could have an interfering effect upon the deeper constitutional treatment. Therefore it is a good idea to first receive approval for self-care.

Course Materials:

The required course materials are as follows:

The Course Syllabus - *Homeopathic Medicine in the Home* (the book you are now reading). This Course Syllabus contains 12 lessons. You will be sending to your instructor the written assignments for every 2 lessons as they are completed. Your written assignments will be corrected and promptly returned to you.

Homeopathic Medicine at Home, by Maesimund B. Panos, M.D., and Jane Heimlich

Materia Medica with Repertory by William Boericke, M.D.

If you are missing either of the above two texts, purchase them immediately from one of the sources for homeopathic books listed in Appendix D, p.134 of this Syllabus; or from Ashwin Publications. As these two texts are required for the course, you must purchase them without delay, in order to be able to proceed.

---

1 Constitutional homeopathic treatment is a form of homeopathic treatment which takes into consideration the totality of a person's symptoms and attributes on the mental, emotional, and physical levels. It can effect a deep balancing in the energetic metabolism of a person, the effects of which can continue to act for months and even years. Under the care of a competent homeopath, a constitutional treatment can deeply improve the level of health, even if one is relatively healthy.

Course Completion Time - Guidelines for a Productive Study

Homeopathic Medicine in the Home consists of 12 lessons. The lessons are structured so that they may be completed at the rate of one lesson per week. Each lesson may be completed in about 7 hours. According to this schedule, the course may be completed in 3 months.

However, you are advised to set your own pace and apply yourself consistently. It is better not to rush through the course. On the other hand, if you proceed too slowly the continuity of learning that builds between the lessons suffers. Therefore, try to maintain a regular study pattern at a comfortable pace. The average completion time for the course ranges between 3-8 months. For the optimal learning experience you are advised to complete the course within 6 months.[1]

Address for Mailing Course Written Assignments:

Ashwins Publications
Post Office Box 1686
Ojai, California 93024

NOTE: If you have not completed and returned an Enrollment/Disclaimer Statement Form, do so now before proceeding to Lesson 1.

---

[1] There will be an extra fee for lessons which are sent in after 14 months from the date of receipt of Course Enrollment/Disclaimer Statement by Ashwins Publications. Maximum course completion time is 3 years.

LESSON 1

The Homeopathic Home Remedy Kit

A homeopathic home remedy kit, available from the homeopathic pharmacies listed below, will make your study of homeopathy a more enjoyable and rewarding experience. Homeopathic home remedy kits offer several advantages:

1. You are given a fairly comprehensive selection of the homeopathic remedies most commonly needed. Having the remedies thus 'at hand,' one is more fully prepared. Remember, homeopathic remedies may not be available in full selection near where you live 24 hours a day.

2. A home remedy kit comes nicely packaged in a convenient carrying case which makes for efficient storage, access, and transport of the remedies.

3. Pharmacies which sell their own home remedy kits offer them at substantially reduced costs from what the remedies normally would cost if purchased individually.

If you do not already have a homeopathic home remedy kit, we encourage you to consider getting one. Since the majority of homeopathic medicines are considered as over-the-counter medicines by the FDA, you can easily order such a remedy kit directly from a homeopathic pharmacy. You do not need to be a doctor to order a homeopathic medicine kit. The following list represents the main sources for homeopathic medicines in the U. S. from which home remedy kits are available.

Note: Make sure any homeopathic home remedy kit which you obtain consists of single homeopathic remedies. Avoid kits consisting of combination homeopathic remedies.

Boericke & Tafel, Inc.
2381 Circadian Way
Santa Rosa, CA 95407
Tel. 1-800-876-9505 (West Coast)
          1-800-272-2820 (East Coast)

Boiron/Borneman
1208 Amosland Rd.
Norwood, PA 19074
Tel. (215) 532-2035 (inside PA)
          1-800-BLU-TUBE (out-of-state)

Dolisos
3014 Rigel Ave.
Las Vegas, Nevada 89103
Tel. (702) 871-7153 (inside Nevada)
          1-800-824-8455 (out-of-state)

Hahnemann Medical Clinic Pharmacy
     (Specify 6c kit)
1918 Bonita Ave.
Berkeley, CA 94704
Tel. (415) 548-5015

Luyties Pharmacal Company
4200 Laclede Avenue
St. Louis, Missouri 63108
Tel. (314) 652-8080 (inside Missouri)
          1-800-325-8080 (out-of-state)

Standard Homeopathic Company
P.O. Box 61067
204-210 West 131st St.
Los Angeles, CA 90061
Tel. 1-800-624-9659

Introduction To The
Course Materials

Let's take a tour of the course books. Throughout the course you will be using these tools in your learning and application of homeopathy.

Homeopathic Medicine in the Home (Syllabus)

This is the Course Syllabus which you are now reading. The Syllabus is both a correspondence course with 12 consecutive lessons and it is a reference work. During the course, should you require clarification on the meaning of a term, you should freely access the Syllabus Glossary on pp. 138-140. If you happen to remain unclear on a meaning, ask your instructor when sending in your written assignments.

Turn now to the Appendices on pp. 129-135. Feel free to access the vital homeopathic resources provided there at any time.

Naturally it is essential that you follow the lessons in order.
However, if the need arises during the course, you should feel some freedom to access information located in lessons you have not yet completed.

Homeopathic Medicine at Home (Text)
by Maesimund B. Panos, M.D., and Jane Heimlich

We will be referring to this book as the TEXT for simplicity's sake. The TEXT contains introductory material on homeopathy and a wealth of practical information for self-care.

Just to familiarize ourselves with the TEXT format let's take a quick look at a chapter. Later we will read this material, so do not read it at this time. But just browse over the chapter on Accidents, pp. 49-79, noticing the material on each injury with accessible charts at the end of the chapter which give a bird's eye view of the accident remedies with their indications for use.

Next turn to p. 246 in the TEXT, Appendix A, "Remedies and Their Abbreviations." There is no need to study this appendix now, we are merely introducing ourselves to this material to know it is there.

Latin names are the internationally accepted scientific standard for all homeopathic remedies. These Latin names can be cumbersome to write out, as well as pronounce. Therefore homeopaths have made abbreviated names and abbreviations for the remedies to make things easier and to save time. Throughout the course we will be referring to this appendix.

Next turn to pp. 249-255 in the TEXT, Appendix B, Mini-Repertory. We will be using this appendix as a tool during our case analysis work. There is no need to read it now.

Next turn to p. 256 in the TEXT, Appendix C, Materia Medica. Again we are just glancing at this appendix to know it is there. This is a simplified and clear listing of some of the main homeopathic remedies with their salient characteristics. This resource is an easy study and referral point.

Boericke's Materia Medica with Repertory
by William Boericke, M.D.

We will be referring to this book as BOERICKE throughout the course. BOERICKE is packed with much information and can take you far in your learning of homeopathy. Do not be put off by the detailed indeces and small print - it is not so difficult to learn to use BOERICKE.

Let's look at BOERICKE now together to get acquainted with it. In the front portion of BOERICKE all of the remedies are listed in alphabetical order with an extensive, yet concise, synopsis of each remedy. Some of the remedy descriptions in BOERICKE are made in medical terminology. While it will not be necessary to learn this terminology in this course, if you are curious or a serious student, the meaning of these terms can usually be found in a medical dictionary and will greatly add to your comprehension.[1] Turn to ARNICA on pp. 76-79 in BOERICKE and then look at ARNICA on p., 258 in the TEXT just to gain the perspective of seeing the greater detail of information in BOERICKE.

Next, let's find two remedy name indeces on pp. 1015-1042 in BOERICKE.[2] These indeces enable you to locate the homeopathic remedy by its common name and latin name.

Let's look together at BOERICKE. Suppose we are trying to locate the plant *Poison Ivy*. Upon alphabetically searching in the front of BOERICKE it cannot be found because the remedies listed in the front of BOERICKE are by their Latin names. Look together with me at *Poison Ivy*, listed on p. 1020 in the Common Name Index as being on p. 552. Turn to p. 552 now in BOERICKE and see the Latin name for *Poison Ivy* - *Rhus toxicodendron*, often referred to as *Rhus tox.* Let's now double check in the TEXT by turning to p. 248, where we see that *Rhus tox.* is the abbreviated name.[3]

WRITTEN ASSIGNMENT

PLEASE USE A SEPARATE SHEET OF PAPER FOR YOUR WRITTEN ASSIGNMENTS THROUGHOUT THE COURSE. INDICATE THE LESSON NUMBER AND THE NUMBER OF THE WRITTEN ASSIGNMENT. WRITE YOUR NAME AND THE DATE OF COMPLETION ON EACH GROUP OF LESSON WRITTEN ASSIGNMENTS YOU RETURN.

1. Here are a few examples for you to try; each of these substances is a widely used remedy. Using the Common Name Index in BOERICKE, p. 1015, and Appendix A in the TEXT, p. 246, find the latin name, abbreviated name and abbreviation for each of the following:

---

1 One example of a medical dictionary is *Taber's Cyclopedic Medical Dictionary* listed in the References section on p. 136 of this Syllabus.
2 Boericke's Materia Medica is published in Indian and non-Indian editions. This Course Syllabus uses the Indian edition. Both Indian and non-Indian editions of Boericke are identical except for some minor differences in the indeces at the back of some non-Indian editions of Boericke. For those students who have a non-Indian edition with these minor differences an explanation will be given for these differences which may be encountered.
3 For practicality's sake, in this Course Syllabus homeopathic medicines will be referred to according to their most commonly used names. In some cases only the first name of the remedy will be recorded, as in the following examples:
Gelsemium sempervirens is commonly known as Gelsemium or Gels. Lycopodium clavatum will be termed Lycopodium or Lyc. Ignatia amara will be called Ignatia or Ign. This is done to simplify things, as there are no other commonly known forms of these remedies with different last names.
   In other cases the full name will be used, as in these examples:
Kali carbonicum is commonly know as Kali carb. or Kali c. We must indicate the second part of the name here to differentiate, as there is more than one form of Kali which is commonly used.

COMFREY

HONEYBEE

YELLOW JASMINE

VEGETABLE CHARCOAL

Turn to pp. 995-1011 in BOERICKE to the Therapeutic Index. This serves as a quick guide pointing one to the most often indicated remedies for a given illness. It is a quick and easy reference point.

From pp. 689-992 in BOERICKE is a detailed index of symptoms known as a Repertory. Here is advanced material we will be using only selectively as beginners.

And on pp. 1-63 in the back of BOERICKE is - Relationship of Remedies and Sides of the Body, which is advanced material that we need not concern ourselves with for the moment.

READING ASSIGNMENT

Read p. 41 in the TEXT: "When and How to Use Your Kit" - the first paragraph. Next: read p. 42 in the TEXT: "Storage."

If you own a homeopathic home remedy kit which has a brochure, browse through it as you would an interesting magazine. Do not try to memorize it. Some things may catch your interest and leave an impression. A complaint you or someone you know has had may bear a resemblance to a remedy description. Through impressions like these we gradually learn the characteristics of the remedies.

Homeopathic Principles and Philosophy

Having familiarized ourselves with the course materials, we are ready to learn about homeopathic principles and philosophy.

Homeopathic Medicine in the Home offers an introduction to the science and art of homeopathy. It is designed to build the skills necessary for resolving common ailments and injuries. The beginner needs a grounding basis of principles from which the sprout of homeopathic knowledge and experience can grow.

The TEXT gives us an introduction to our study. Historical perspectives on the origin and development of homeopathy, and its basic principles are explored.

Read pp. 5-14 in the TEXT, stopping at the Comparison of Homeopathy and Allopathy.

WRITTEN ASSIGNMENT

2. *Explain the Law of Similars in your own words.*

3. *In the homeopathic materia medica are listed characteristic symptoms for each of the remedies. From what source are these symptoms derived? How does the materia medica get its information?*

4. *Homeopathic medicines are non-toxic and cause no side effects. Why is this so?*

5. *Why do most homeopaths usually give only one remedy at a time?*

Homeopathy - An Energetic Explanation

Homeopathy is an energy medicine. A fuller understanding of homeopathic pharmacology helps us to grasp the energetic concept.

Homeopathic medicines are prepared (as mentioned on p. 12 TEXT) through a process known as potentization, where the original substance is diluted and succussed. Remedies in the United States are commonly available in 'X' and 'C' potencies.

Take the example of a homeopathic remedy labelled - Nux vomica 6X. The '6X' refers to the potency of the remedy. The 'X' indicates that the Nux vomica has been diluted 1 part to 9 parts diluting medium. 'X' potencies are known as decimal potencies. If a remedy is labelled 6X it means that one part of the original material substance of the remedy has been added to 9 parts diluting medium and succussed (shaken). Then one part of the resulting solution is added to another 9 parts diluting solution and succussed. This process is carried out 6 times to arrive at the 6X potency.[1]

If a remedy is labelled Nux vomica 6C, it means that the potency is on the 'C' or centesimal scale. 'C' potencies are diluted 1 part original substance to 99 parts diluting medium. A remedy of 6C potency has been diluted one part original substance to 99 parts diluting medium and succussed. Then one part of the resulting solution is added to another 99 parts diluting medium and succussed. This process is carried out 6 times to arrive at the 6C potency. If a remedy is labelled Nux vomica 6 - just the number without an X or a C following it - this means that automatically it is a 'C' potency and would be Nux vomica 6C in this case.

'C' potencies are more diluted than 'X' potencies. 6C is more diluted than 6X. The higher one goes in diluted potency, the more powerful the remedy becomes energetically. Therefore the 6C potency is generally considered more powerful than the 6X potency, from an energetic perspective.

---

1 Once a homeopathic remedy is thus prepared in its liquid form, known as a liquid dilution, drops of this liquid dilution are then usually placed onto sugar pellets in individual bottles for dispensing to the public.

If you have access to both 'X' and 'C' potencies you may be confused as to their equivalent values. For example a 6X potency is approximately equivalent to a 3C potency. They are not exactly the same, because they have been succussed a different number of times, but they have the same amount of dilution. The approximate equivalent of a 6C potency would be 12X. So if you have an 'X' potency and want to know its approximate equivalent value in 'C' potency divide by 2. If you have a 'C' potency and would like to know its approximate value in the 'X' potency then multiply by 2.

In any homeopathic remedy having a potency of at least or higher than, 12C or 24X, there is not a physical trace of the original substance remaining. Yet as one goes higher in diluted potency the remedy becomes even more potent. High potency remedies, generally considered higher than 30C, can act deeply and powerfully on the personality and physical nature. It is as if, through the process of potentization, the remedy is freed from its material form and the representative etheric energy that is behind the substance in the material creation is freed to interact with the patient's energy field.

In illustrating the energetic action of a homeopathic remedy, we use the term *vital force* to indicate the energy of a person's health. Western medicine's *immunological defense mechanism* and the *chi* of Eastern medicine are synonymous with the concept of the *vital force.* Let us now take an example to show the action of a homeopathic remedy:

A person who has insomnia from having been overjoyed upon receiving good news. He wants to sleep but cannot get his restless nervous system to turn down. His mind is active and clear. He is wide awake yet knows he needs to rise early the next day.

There is a remedy in homeopathy - Coffea cruda - which is derived from unroasted coffee beans and is commonly known as Coffea. Coffea can cause symptoms of insomnia (identical to the experience of the person described above) in a healthy person.

READING ASSIGNMENT

Turn to Coffea in BOERICKE, pp. 222-224, and read the first paragraph, together with the section Mind and Sleep. This is a detailed account of the symptoms which the remedy can cause in a healthy person. The detailed account of symptoms is taken from a proving as is described on p. 11 of the TEXT.

Getting back to the person with insomnia - his vital force is not quite able on its own to throw off the insomnia and nervous excitability. Then he is given the homeopathic remedy Coffea. What happens? Here is an energetic explanation.

The remedy Coffea is taken and the energy of the remedy resonates in similarity with the existing state of imbalance being experienced.

Because the remedy Coffea was taken and came from the outside, *the vital force* of the person is provoked to throw off the energy of the remedy Coffea. The *vital force* is able to do this and this process occurs automatically. But what happens is that in throwing off the energy of the remedy, the existing imbalance which matched the energy of the remedy is also thrown off. The imbalance is cleared and sleep is effortlessly attained.

We now see that homeopathy acts by stimulating the *vital force* or *immunological defense mechanism*. In doing so, not only is the complaint removed but one becomes healthier in the process.

READING ASSIGNMENT

To further explore the principles of homeopathy in relation to other therapies and receive perspectives on the status and direction of homeopathy in the U.S. and the world today: Read pp. 14-21 in the TEXT. Then browse through Appendix B of this Syllabus on pp. 130-131, which details resources of homeopathic organizations and in-person trainings.

WRITTEN ASSIGNMENT

6. Homeopathy views all symptoms - Mental, Emotional, and Physical - as part of an interrelated whole. How does the approach of standard medicine differ?

Deeper Dimensions of Homeopathy

This information will serve to educate those students who wish to undergo a chronic constitutional homeopathic treatment under the care of an experienced homeopath.[1] It will also be useful to those in the healing arts who are considering a deeper study of homeopathy, and gaining further understandings of the natural laws of healing.

Homeopathic medicines, because they are energetic, can act deeply on a person's energy affecting the strata of personality and the physical nature. Properly used, homeopathy can serve to effect deep balances in the energetic metabolism of a person. Homeopathy can serve as a tool to assist man's consciousness to achieve a greater sense of mastery amidst life's challenges. Inherited predispositions to illness can be removed. Applied in this way, homeopathy could enable parents to bring a healthier generation into the world.

Since homeopathic medicines can have a profound effect upon the human organism, it is important to deeply understand what constitutes health on the Mental, Emotional, and Physical planes of the human being. Also a perspective is needed into the dynamic interrelationships between the Mental, Emotional, and Physical levels which function as a totality. And we need an understanding of the natural laws of healing that act through these levels. Contemporary homeopathy has received much knowledge and insight in these areas from the contributions of master homeopath George Vithoulkas.

---

1 Appendix E of the Syllabus on p. 135 provides guidelines for locating and selecting a competent homeopathic physician or practitioner, if you do not already have one.

Health on the Mental, Emotional, and Physical planes may be defined as follows:

Mental Plane

". . . on this level are the functions most crucial to the expression of the individual as a human being."[1]

There are 3 indispensable qualities upon which health on the mental plane is gauged. They are:

" 1. Clarity
2. Rationality, coherence and logical sequence
3. Creative service for the good of others as well as for the good of oneself."[2]

These 3 qualities must all be present together in order to have true mental health. For example, ". . . the master criminal who is highly intelligent and plans a theft or a murder with the utmost degree of clarity and rationality of thinking. Yet this person is ill in the deepest regions of his being, because he is pursuing selfish goals at the expense of other people. Such a mentality pervades our modern world to an extreme degree, and is a root cause of the problems of competition, violence, alcohol and drug abuse, poverty, and war."[3] Thus we see the importance of unselfishness in true mental sanity.

Emotional Plane

The next level in importance is the emotional plane. "At the highest state of emotional health, the individual experiences an absolute dynamic calmness combined with love for self, others, and environment."[4] In this state of emotional well being one is free from such negative emotional passions as anger, anxiety, fear, hatred, jealousy, and depression. There is an active interplay of positive emotions with the outside world creating a sense of unity.

Physical Plane

Health on the physical plane is a high level of well-being where there is ". . . experienced complete freedom of body functions, when none of the organs are limited and when there is no sense of negative awareness of the body."[5] In this state a person is free from disease and physical limitation from having to put too much attention on the body. In this state there is an independence from undue reliance on drugs, special diets or other therapies to maintain health.

---

1 George Vithoulkas, *The Science of Homeopathy* (New York: Grove Press, 1980), p.23
2 *Ibid.*, p. 27
3 *Ibid.*, p. 28
4 Ibid., p. 31-32
5 *Ibid.*, p. 40

The Hierarchy of Health

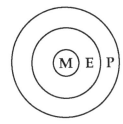

M=Mental

E=Emotional

P=Physical[1]

In the hierarchy of health, as the above diagram illustrates, the general idea is that the mental plane represents the deepest level of health. The emotional plane is next in importance and the physical plane, although important, is more on the periphery of the organism.

Generally we can say that a person can be in good physical health, yet if that person is deeply depressed emotionally and is in a state of mental confusion - this is a deeper level of suffering. This person is the most seriously ill. On the other hand, a person confined to a wheel chair who is emotionally happy and healthy in the sphere of the mind may experience joy, write a book, or creatively express him- or herself in many ways. Naturally, however, our goal is to enjoy optimum health on all levels.

The following schema, developed by George Vithoulkas, shows the gradation of depth of illness within each of the planes.

Mental	Emotional	Physical
Complete Mental Confusion	Suicidal Depression	Brain ailments
Destructive Delirium	Apathy	Heart ailments
Paranoid Ideas	Sadness	Endocrine ailments
Delusions	Anguish	Liver ailments
Lethargy	Phobias	Lung ailments
Dullness	Anxiety	Kidney ailments
Lack of Concentration	Irritability	Bone ailments
Forgetfulness	Dissatisfaction	Muscle ailments
Absent-mindedness		Skin ailments [2]

On the mental level we see complaints ranging from minor absentmindedness to delusions and finally complete mental confusion being the most serious.
We see emotional complaints ranging from minor dissatisfaction to suicidal depression.
On the physical level, complaints on the skin are less serious than complaints of the vital organs and nervous system.

Note that a minor mental weakness such as absentmindedness is of course less serious than a serious emotional complaint such as suicidal depression. And a minor emotional condition such as irritability is of course less serious than one of the most serious physical diseases such as brain cancer. Thus we must understand that there is an overlap between these symptoms on the various planes of being.

---

1 *Ibid.*, p. 24
2 *Ibid.*

Hering's Laws of Cure [1]

The 3 planes of health - mental, emotional, and physical - have a dynamic interrelationship which is explained by Hering's Laws of Cure. Hering's Laws of cure are natural laws of healing which are observable in homeopathy and in other forms of holistic healing. They state that healing occurs at the deepest levels first and proceeds through to less serious levels toward the periphery - the physical plane.[2]

On the physical level, cure proceeds in the direction of going from the nervous system and vital organs to the skin and on the skin going from the head to the feet. Previously experienced ailments reappear and then disappear starting from the most recent going back in time chronologically. Is that a little confusing? Just read the following example to clarify the point.

A man has delusions that he is a criminal. At the same time he is deeply depressed. So we see he is ill mentally and emotionally. Physically he is all right, although he has had asthmatic type breathing during the hay fever season. As a child, he had a case of psoriasis, a skin complaint. The patient is given the *Similimum;* the remedy which matches the totality of the patient's symptoms. In response to the remedy, the man's delusions (on the mental level) disappear first. His emotional depression then lifts and he feels healthy internally. Even though it is not hay fever season, the man develops a bout of asthma which lasts for a week. As the asthma is starting to fade, the man develops a bad case of psoriasis over his entire body. Over a period of 6 months the psoriasis gradually clears up, starting first at the head and proceeding downwards until it leaves at the feet.

Thus we see how cure begins at deeper levels and can proceed towards the skin, finally leaving at the feet, in many chronic cases.

Perspective on Suppression

Understanding Hering's laws of natural healing offers discriminating insights into the nature of true healing. This is of special importance in the treatment of chronic long standing conditions.

As an example, suppose a person has been relatively healthy mentally, emotionally, and physically, yet has had a chronic skin problem of warts. Suppose the warts had been 'successfully' removed with laser surgery and the warts did not return. This kind of therapy does not remove the cause of the warts, however. Now, instead of warts the person has developed arthritis, along with a much lower threshold of irritability. Thus the disease, which manifested as warts, is driven deeper into the organism. This is known as suppression. Now we see the person suffers from a more serious physical ailment and is weaker emotionally. The person then receives corticosteroid medications, which appear to remove the symptoms of the arthritis. As a result of this suppressive treatment the person now develops heart disease, along with a violent temper and periods of deep depression.

Through this example we observe how suppressive treatments cause the illness to be driven into deeper levels of health and we observe the person's health deteriorating.

---

1 Constantine Hering M.D. was one of the great nineteenth century homeopaths. He is known for his role in bringing homeopathy to America from Germany in the early 1800's. Dr. Hering observed and defined these laws of cure which now bear his name.
2 This generally assumes that the physical complaint, which manifests as part of the healing process, is not seriously life threatening.

We see, therefore, that understanding the levels of health and their hierarchy in the light of Hering's Laws of Cure provides important insights into the nature of what constitutes true healing. It is especially important to keep these perspectives in mind when choosing your own health care and in knowing whether your health is improving.

WRITTEN ASSIGNMENT

7. A child once had terrible reactions to milk and eggs, causing diarrhea. Now the mother has a strict diet for the child, avoiding these foods. The child is not suffering from any diarrhea as long as the diet is adhered to. According to the definition of health, is the child healthy? Why?

8. According to the hierarchy of health in homeopathy - which complaint is more serious: a deep depression or a skin eczema covering most of the body? Why?

READING ASSIGNMENT

Maesimund Panos, M.D., shares with us her work with homeopathy from an experiential view. This perspective further educates us as to how a homeopath works in a deeper constitutional way.

Read Chapter 2 in the TEXT - pp. 22-32.

Here is the official definition and explanation of homeopathy as given by the Homeopathic Pharmacopeia of the U.S.; it confirms what we have covered thus far. (Note - The Homeopathic Pharmacopeia of the U.S., known as HPUS, is the text which standardizes the manufacture of homeopathic remedies.)

"Homeopathy/Homeotherapeutics, a unique medical specialty, is concerned with the whole or total patient, whose disorder or disease is expressed by a complex of symptoms or syndrome which involves both psyche or soma, i.e., emotional and/or mental as well as physical symptoms. Philosophically, it is based on the Principle of Similars, 'Similia Similibus Curentur,' (likes cures likes), i.e., a substance which is capable of evoking certain symptoms in an essentially healthy human being under controlled research procedures, may become a potentially therapeutic agent when prepared according to the specifications of the Homeopathic Pharmacopeia and prescribed in accordance with homeopathic standards."

NOTE: When you have completed the <u>eight</u> written assignments for this lesson, put them aside in a safe place, together with any questions you might have about the material, and continue with lesson 2. When you have completed the written assignments for that lesson, you will be instructed to send to your instructor the work you have completed for lessons one <u>and</u> two. You will then continue through the course in this manner, sending in two assignments at a time, at the end of each *even-numbered lesson*. The address for mailing in your written assignments is given on p. 2 of this Syllabus.

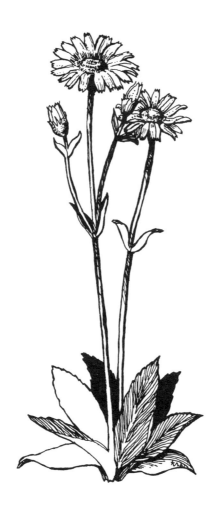

Arnica montana (Leopard's Bane)

LESSON 2

We are about ready to begin the practical use of homeopathy. Here are some practical considerations for taking homeopathic remedies.

A Word About Taking Homeopathic Remedies

Depending upon the pharmacy where you obtain your remedies, they will come either in milk sugar (lactose) tablets or cane sugar (sucrose) pellets. The sucrose pellets are available in a tiny almost granular #10 size going up in diameter to the larger spherical #40 pill size. The lactose tablets are easier to administer to infants and pets, since they are composed of a softer sugar which can be crushed and dissolved more rapidly. The tiny #10 pellets are also good for infants and pets, as their small size renders them quickly dissolvable.

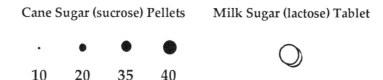

Cane Sugar (sucrose) Pellets   Milk Sugar (lactose) Tablet

10   20   35   40

The most commonly seen sizes (actual) of homeopathic sucrose pellets, compared to the softer lactose tablet.

Follow the instructions given on your remedy vial or bottle as to the amount which constitutes a dose. When taking homeopathic remedies tap the required amount of pellets or tablets into the cap of the remedy container and empty the contents onto the tongue. Dissolve in mouth. Avoid touching the remedy. If any of the remedy falls on the floor, etc., do not replace it into the container, rather discard it. If too much of the remedy comes into the cap, gently tap some of it back into the container without touching it. The remedies should be taken in a clean mouth, free from food, mints, toothpaste, tobacco, etc. Generally speaking it is better to take a homeopathic remedy at least 15 minutes before eating or 30 minutes after eating.

If you are ever in a situation of running low on a remedy while not having immediate access to get more, such as a weekend evening, it is all right to take less of the remedy than the recommended amount. It is not so important whether one takes 5 pellets or 1 or 2. The effect should be the same. As long as the mouth is clean, the remedy will be viable. This is so because homeopathic medicines are in an energetic form - they are not in the physical material form of the remedy. So whether we take 3 pellets or 30, the energetic value should be the same.

There may be a few rare instances when someone has a severe reaction to even minute quantities of sugar. How could this person take a homeopathic remedy? First of all, it should be understood that this person should go to an experienced homeopath for deeper homeopathic treatment. In most situations it is not at all difficult for a homeopath to remove this reaction to sugar and raise the person's level of health. Homeopathic medicines are, however, available in liquid form consisting of about 80% purified water and 20% ethyl alcohol. These liquid remedies are available from most homeopathic pharmacies.

Recommended Frequency of Usage

Frequency of usage is a matter which is individualized to suit the circumstances.

The general rule is - give as needed. In the beginning of an illness or when treating an injury it may be necessary to repeat the remedy with maximum frequency. Generally, the maximum frequency for the repetition of the remedy is indicated in most remedy kit brochures and on your remedy vials.

With improvement, the frequency of usage can be reduced as the need decreases. The general recommended guidelines for frequency of usage *after* the most severe stages of the complaint have passed are these:

For potencies 3C, 6C, and 3X, 6X, 12X; give 3 times a day.

For potencies 12C and 30X; give 2 times per day.

For potency 30C; give one time per day.[1] Generally, as a rule, 30C is not repeated for more than a few days. However, this is not a 'hard and fast' rule; there may be exceptions.

Generally speaking a higher potency will act longer and require less repetition than a lower potency. For example, suppose you have the remedy Arnica in 3C and 30C potencies. In a given case where 3C might initially need repetition every hour, Arnica in 30C potency may produce a similar result if repeated every 12 hours.

Discontinue when improvement is well established.

IMPORTANT NOTE: The beginner in homeopathy is advised, as a rule, to refrain from using higher potencies of homeopathic remedies, such as 200C. Homeopathic remedies with potencies ranging in ascending strength from 1M (which is the equivalent of 1000C) going up to 10M, 50M, and CM are extremely high in energetic potency. The beginning student of homeopathy should definitely avoid using these highest potencies.

READING ASSIGNMENT

Read text pp. 40-43 starting with the paragraph in the middle of p. 40 and stopping at the end of Storage. Read pp. 47-48: The Combination Game.

Homeopathy for Accidents and Injuries

We begin with the practical use of homeopathy for accidents and injuries. It is easy to find the right remedy for injuries because usually there is only a handful of remedies that need to be considered for any given injury. Also there are few differentiating details that need to be considered, and the remedies are often specific for certain kinds of injuries.

---

1 The recommended frequency of usage for 30C in Emotional Complaints is different and is given in Lesson 10, p. 104 of this Syllabus.

Injuries can respond dramatically to homeopathy because recovery depends on the organism's recuperative powers and homeopathy precisely activates these powers. This builds the beginner's confidence in the homeopathic science and in one's own homeopathic abilities. Just about every homeopath has 'miracle stories' regarding the homeopathic resolution of injuries, and I will not be in the least surprised if you also experience some.

Throughout the TEXT, mention will be made of those conditions which warrant professional help. Even in those situations homeopathy can often help alleviate the suffering and speed the recovery and healing process as an adjunct to licensed medical help. One precaution needed with regard to injuries is that in cases of broken bones, or where broken bones are suspected, Symphytum should not be given until the bones are set in the correct position, because it stimulates the union of bone so rapidly.

A Word About Frequency of Usage For Accidents and Injuries

The general guidelines to follow are basically those given by the TEXT for accidents and injuries: 3-5 pellets 3 or 4 times a day, or when pain is severe every 30 minutes to 1 hour as needed. Decrease frequency of usage as improvement is seen. Discontinue when improvement is well established.

Sometimes injury situations are unique and the frequency of usage is adjusted to suit the conditions. Here the question of how often to repeat a homeopathic medicine ultimately rests in the hands of yourself or your homeopath.

A Word About Diluting Tinctures to Make Lotions

In the material we are about to cover, lotions are made from tinctures (which are found in most remedy kits) for external application. The recommended and easy way to prepare a lotion, in any quantity desired, is to dilute one part tincture to 4 parts water. This will help take the sting out of the tincture due to its high alcohol content. Prepare your lotion in an empty one ounce dropper bottle, which is readily obtainable at most drug stores. The dropper is a convenient means of dispensing lotions. For maximum shelf life store the lotion in the refrigerator when not in use. Otherwise, because the alcohol content has been lowered, the lotion may eventually spoil and turn brackish at room temperature.

READING ASSIGNMENT

Read pp. 49-52 in the TEXT: Bruises (Contusions). Then turn to the Materia Medica in the TEXT and read the remedies Arnica, Hypericum, Ledum, and Ruta.

Please add the following information about Hypericum to the TEXT Materia Medica by neatly printing it into the TEXT or adding it to your notes:

Hypericum: *specific for automobile whiplash injuries, especially when there are shooting pains and / or sensations of numbness or tingling.*

WRITTEN ASSIGNMENT

1. A child falls down concrete steps and is generally bruised all over. The child's shin was bumped and scraped badly during the fall and the skin is broken there.

Which remedy would one most likely think of giving the child first internally? Why?

What might be a good lotion to use for dressing the broken skin on the child? Why?

What remedy may come to mind as a second choice in the event that the shin remains painful?

2. A man gets his fingernail closed in a door jamb (ouch!).

Another man slips while ice skating and lands on his tail bone.

Another man has shooting pains going from the neck to the elbow since an automobile whiplash accident.

What one injury-specific remedy comes to mind for these injuries?

3. What remedy may be indicated for a black eye where Arnica fails to heal and the victim feels better by putting cold compresses on it?

READING ASSIGNMENT

Read in the TEXT pp. 53-55, "Strains and Sprains." Then go on to read the Materia Medica for Rhus tox. and Symphytum given below:

Rhus toxicodendron / Rhus tox.

Indicated for trauma to tendons, ligaments, connective tissue.
Pulled muscles.
Strained lower back from lifting.
Muscular tension, stiffness of muscles and joints.
Pain is worse after having been sitting or at rest, and when just in the act of rising from the resting position - pain is worse. Pain gets better through continued movement and stretching.

       WORSE FROM (<)
              <first movement when rising
              <cold wet weather

       BETTER FROM (>)
              >hot baths
              >warm dry weather
              >massage
              >continued movement

Note the use of the symbols > and <.

> indicates improved by, made better from, or ameliorated by.

< indicates made worse from or aggravated by.

Get into the habit of using these symbols in your written assignments and in your homeopathic work. It will save a little time. For example, if someone says he or she feels worse from cold wet weather, we can write <cold wet weather.

Symphytum / Symph. (Comfrey - Knitbone)

Stimulates the rapid union of bones and healing of ligaments and tendons.
The best remedy for traumatic injuries to the eyeball from blunt objects.
Indicated for injuries to the tailbone (coccyx) where Hypericum fails to help.
Indicated for injuries to the lining of the shin bone (periosteum) where Ruta fails to help.
Indicated for automobile whiplash injuries where Hypericum fails to help.
One should be sure the bones are set in the right place before giving Symphytum.

As you can see, in many varieties of physical trauma, Arnica is often indicated first. Arnica activates the body's energies to recover from the trauma. Many times there will be a specific injury along with the general trauma. In these cases, after giving Arnica there may be some improvement generally. However, where the signs clearly indicate there has been specific injury which was not alleviated by the Arnica, then we give another remedy which matches the specific tissue damage. An example of this is Dr. Panos's description of her wrenched ankle on p. 54.

In these cases - when the injury is *unresolved* by Arnica - this might become apparent within an hour after taking the Arnica. In such urgent situations the second remedy may be needed *without delay.* With Dr. Panos's case, she waited a day. Other situations may warrant taking the second remedy sooner.

WRITTEN ASSIGNMENT

4. After the first big winter snow storm, the father of the house, who has a sedentary desk job, strains his lower back shoveling snow. The next day he feels pain, stiffness, and is better from hot baths and having Lucy, his wife, massage his back.

What remedy shall we think to give father and why?

IMPORTANT NOTE: If father is being rubbed with an aromatic muscle linament, the linament would need to be discontinued in order to be assured the remedy will act. Also, one should never store or open up a homeopathic remedy vial in the presence of such aromatic vapors. The camphor and menthol in the linament can antidote the action of a homeopathic medicine.

Electric blankets also can antidote the action of a homeopathic remedy, and they disrupt the energy in the body - thus are unhealthy.

Ultra sound therapy, which is used by chiropractors and physical therapists, has also been known to antidote homeopathic remedies.

Guidelines for Studying Homeopathic Medicines - Materica Medica

Each homeopathic medicine has its own unique properties and detailed characteristics, which are known as Materia Medica. The reference books which contain this information are known as Materia Medicas. In our study of Materia Medica we come to realize that for each homeopathic medicine there is a lengthy and intricate description. It seems overwhelming and impossible to remember all these details. Fortunately it is unnecessary to memorize everything. We do, however, need to make efforts to become familiar with the most outstanding aspects of the commonly used homeopathic medicines. These aspects are known as Keynotes. The Materia Medica Written Assignments which follow in this Syllabus emphasize the salient aspects (keynotes) of each homeopathic medicine.

The study of Materia Medica can be supported by your practical experience in applying homeopathic skills to resolve minor ailments. These remedies which we become familiar with through experience tend to make an indelible impression. These impressions are well earned gifts which remain in our memories.

In beginning our study of homeopathic medicines, emphasis is placed on the following aspects:

> The Sphere of Action of a Remedy
> Sensations
> Modalities
> General Symptoms
> Mental / Emotional State

- **The Sphere of Action of a Remedy:**
  Each homeopathic medicine may have its own sphere of action. When prominent, the sphere of action is worthwhile to remember. For example - Rhus tox. has a sphere of action involving tendons, ligaments, connective tissue, and the skin.

- **Sensations:**
  These are sensations of pain or discomfort, such as aching, burning, itching, and pulsating, etc. For example, Belladonna is known to have pulsating pains.

- **Modalities:**
  These are conditions by which the symptoms are improved or aggravated. For example - Bryonia's pain is *worse from movement and warmth*. The pains of Rhus tox. are *improved by movement and warmth*.

- **General Symptoms:**
  This refers to the general body warmth or chilliness, the degree of thirst or thirstlessness, food cravings or aversions, perspiration, appearance of the skin, and the general energy level. For example, Arsenicum album is generally known to be chilly.[1] Pulsatilla is generally known to be thirstless. Nux vomica is generally known to desire spicy foods. Phosphorus is generally known to be thirsty for cold drinks. Belladonna is generally known to have a red flushed face. And Gelsemium is generally known to be dull and listless.

---

1 Note - Attributes or symptoms which call for a particular remedy are discussed at places in this Syllabus, being given the name of the homeopathic medicine which applies. Thus: "Arsenicum album is generally known to be chilly" may be understood as - chilliness is an attribute characteristic of the homeopathic medicine, Arsenicum album.

• **Mental / Emotional State**
    Some illustrative examples of this are the irritability of Bryonia, the weepy changeable moods of Pulsatilla, and the fearful anxiety of Aconite.

These are the most notable aspects we focus on in our study of Materia Medica. However, homeopathic medicines have a great variety of attributes, and with any given remedy there could be other important aspects. An example of this is the remedy Pulsatilla, which is well known for its thick yellow mucus. So we see that Discharges from the body can also be a notable aspect of focus in certain remedies. As we study homeopathic medicines and become familiar with them we learn to develop a sense of what is important to remember about each particular remedy. The Materia Medica Written Assignments in this Syllabus are designed to emphasize these most important aspects of each remedy.

If it still seems that there will be too much memorization involved in learning the keynotes of the common homeopathic medicines 'remember' that you do not have to memorize it all. The TEXT Materia Medica and BOERICKE are at your disposal to look up this information. In summary, it is through continued application of homeopathy in practical experiential situations, coupled with study, that we become familiar with the keynote characteristics of the commonly used remedies. What is learned in this manner is remembered with ease and may be looked upon as an investment which will serve you many times over in the future.

Moreover, there is a great advantage in our learning of Materia Medica in that practically all of the remedies have multiple uses. For example, the remedy Rhus tox. is useful for muscular strains, but it is also useful in cases of the flu, and in shingles - a form of herpes. The good news in our learning of Materia Medica is that the main keynotes - i.e., Sensations, Modalities, General Symptoms and Mental / Emotional State, which are characteristic to a homeopathic remedy - usually remain the SAME for ALL the illnesses that the remedy can cure.

With the remedy Rhus tox. the pains resulting from a muscular strain typically are aching and are accompanied by a stiffness which is worse in cold wet weather. The flu and shingles of Rhus tox. are also worse in cold wet weather.

Nausea, nosebleed, headaches, and cough are all ailments which can be resolved by Phosphorus when the symptoms point to Phosphorus. In each of these complaints the Phosphorus case would commonly have the keynote symptom of an above average thirst for cold drinks.

Conjunctivitis (an inflammation of the mucous membrane lining the eyelids), a head cold, an upset stomach, and painful menstruation are among a few of the many complaints which can be resolved by Pulsatilla when the symptoms match Pulsatilla. In each of these complaints usually one finds an element of being easily moved to tears, or of desiring company and affection.

Therefore as we will be studying the different minor ailments and the most often indicated homeopathic medicines for them, the same medicines which we will have read about for other complaints will keep cropping up. Again and again we will be reading the same characteristic keynotes for each medicine. This facilitates and simplifies our learning of Materia Medica.

The following illustration shows how one homeopathic remedy can resolve many illnesses while the keynotes of the remedy remain the same.

Pulsatilla can cure many illnesses when the symptoms correspond to Pulsatilla. In each of these different illnesses which may require Pulsatilla the characteristic keynotes of Pulsatilla will, as a rule, remain the same. [1]

Arthritis

Cystitis - Inflammation of the bladder

Painful Breasts

Bronchitis

Ear Infections

Hemorrhoids

Heart Palpitations

Indigestion

Absense of menses

Irregular menses

Pre-menstrual syndrome

Mumps

German measles

Obesity

Sciatica

Varicose veins

Colds

Conjunctivitis - inflammation of mucous membrane inside eyelids.

Cough

Diarrhea

Painful menses

Prostate problems

KEYNOTES OF PULSATILLA

- **SENSATIONS:**
  Pains shifting and changing from one location to another.

- **MODALITIES:**
  Worse from heat, in a warm room, from warm applications. worse fatty food, hot foods.
  better cool open air, cold applications, cold food and drink.

- **DISCHARGES** - thick yellow mucus, easily expectorated/ profuse, bland, non- irritating.

- **GENERAL SYMPTOMS:**
  Warm blooded
  Thirstlessness
  Desires cold foods

- **MENTAL / EMOTIONAL STATE:**
  Emotional; weeping easily
  Desires affection and attention and feels better from it.
  Changeable moods.

[1] Note that in any given illness requiring a given remedy, one does not expect to see **all** of the keynote characteristics of the remedy present. Usually in actual experience, one just sees a few of the keynotes. This process is further explained later on in the course Lesson 7, Prescribing Hint #1, p. 70.

Answering Your Materia Medica Written Assignments

Throughout the course we will be learning the most outstanding traits of the commonly used homeopathic medicines for self-care, in the Materia Medica Written Assignments. Before starting each series of Materia Medica Written Assignments, be sure to first write on your answer paper the name of the Remedy being studied, with the words Materia Medica. In the following Written Assignment therefore, before completing answers 5 through 11 which pertain to Bryonia alba, write <u>Bryonia alba Materia Medica</u> on your paper. This will serve to make the answers more understandable when referring back to them, and your instructor's comments and corrections will then be more meaningful.

READING ASSIGNMENT

Bryonia alba Materia Medica.
Read Bryonia alba in the TEXT materia medica on p. 260 and, if available, in your remedy kit brochure. Read Bryonia alba in BOERICKE on pp. 132-135, scanning the material by placing emphasis on finding the same symptoms in the TEXT. Read the modalities carefully.

WRITTEN ASSIGNMENT

Bryonia alba Materia Medica.
5. *What is the classic modality that makes a Bryonia state worse?*

6. *Describe the Bryonia thirst, and the temperature of drink that is desired.*

7. *Describe the state of Bryonia mucus membranes.*

8. *What is the mood of the Bryonia patient?*

9. *What is the pain that typifies Bryonia?*

10. *What temperature improves Bryonia?*

11. *Write the abbreviation for Bryonia.*

READING ASSIGNMENT

Read p. 65, "Sports Injuries," in TEXT and look over pp. 75-79 - Sports Injuries Chart.

Cuprum metallicum / Cuprum / Cupr. is a remedy that may be indicated in sports injuries. Cuprum is an important remedy for cramps in the calves and soles of the feet, as well as the palms. Imagine some situations which would cause such cramps and know that Cuprum could likely provide immediate relief. If you look at Cuprum in BOERICKE you will see it is also an epilepsy remedy, but epilepsy is an illness only the experienced homeopathic physician should treat.

Anyone who has taken up a new physical activity knows what it is like to be afflicted the day afterward with the bruised sore aching feeling in muscles and joints that often ensues. In the 'Sports Injuries Chart' on p. 77 of the TEXT Arnica is rightly given as the remedy for this condition. However if Arnica does not relieve, there are other homeopathic remedies which may make a big difference.

Sarcolacticum acidum / Sarcol ac., is a homeopathic remedy derived from sarcolactic acid. It can be a valuable remedy where Arnica fails to relieve. Sarcolactic acid is found in muscles as a by product of physical exertion. The key symptoms to remember for Sarcolactum acidum are:

> Sore aching pains and stiffness in muscles, joints, and bones.
> General feelings of weakness in the limbs.
> Aversion to exercise.
> The pains are worse from movement.

When Arnica has failed to relieve and these symptoms are present, Sarcolacticum acidum is recommended in the 6C or 12X potency. It should provide relief.

If, however, there is soreness, aching, and stiffness remaining after Arnica and the pains are *better* from movement and stretching we would be inclined to give Rhus tox.

Wounds, Insect Stings, Bites and Burns

Petroleum based ointments of Arnica and Calendula are in most remedy kits. Remember never to apply the Arnica ointment to broken skin, as it is known to cause festering blisterlike eruptions.

In handling burns, it is best to avoid applying petroleum based ointments. The lotions of Calendula or Hypercum may be used in cases where skin is broken and in handling burns as an external wash or dressing. To make a lotion, dilute one part tincture to 4 parts water.

Most wounds heal best with air, and the petroleum based Calendula ointment cuts off air to the wound. Therefore, Calendula and Hypericum lotions are recommended for wounds, as they promote optimal healing by letting air in. Calendula ointment is excellent for applications on chafed skin, diaper rash, and minor abrasions.

READING ASSIGNMENT

In the TEXT read pp. 55-59 on Wounds.

NOTE: For puncture wounds, in addition to Ledum tincture used externally as described in the text on pp. 58 and 59, the homeopathic remedy Ledum may serve well in these cases if taken internally.

READING ASSIGNMENT

In the TEXT read pp. 59-62.

Take note of Dr. Panos's experience with her daughter's yellow jacket stings, illustrating how often to repeat a remedy. Ledum was given in repeated doses spontaneously in response to the swelling and inflammation of the immediate situation.

Also note that Ledum is indicated internally in cases of bites from poisonous spiders and scorpions. Ledum is specific for bites and stings that are venomous and for puncture wounds with swelling, soreness, and eccymosis (black and blue discoloration). If Ledum can be given quite soon after the sting or bite it may abort or minimize other side effects from the sting or bite that otherwise would have occurred. In the author's own experience there have been two instances of scorpion bite in which the person was given Ledum immediately after the bite. In both instances there was minimized discomfort and rapid recovery. If you are exposed to encounters with these creatures you may wish to order the extra remedies the TEXT indicates, to have them on hand. The remedies the TEXT mentions are indicated for more serious symptoms following a bite or sting. These could be taken hopefully while on the way to the hospital. You are advised to follow the Beyond First Aid advice throughout the TEXT.

READING ASSIGNMENT

Read pp. 62-64 in the TEXT - Burns. Read Cantharis in the TEXT - materia medica.

WRITTEN ASSIGNMENT

12. A woman burns her hand on the stove. What relief might the taking of Cantharis bring?

Finding Injuries In Boericke

If you ever come across an injury that is not in the TEXT, or if you are searching for more information about the use of homeopathy for an injury, in order to successfully select the right remedy you will need to become more familiar with the use of BOERICKE.

Turn to p. 963 in BOERICKE and find 'Injuries'. Glance over all the categories of injuries listed followed by the remedies indicated for that injury. Note the remedies are abbreviated and you should have no trouble finding an abbreviated remedy by looking it up in the front of BOERICKE, going alphabetically by the abbreviation. The remedies listed in this index are in both plain type and italics. The remedies in italics are more strongly indicated for the injury. By referring to the detailed materia medica in the front of BOERICKE, we can study the indicated remedies for that injury in order to select the best one. In most cases, however, the material in the TEXT will be sufficient.

Emergencies

As with the application of homeopathy in accidents and injuries, emergency use of homeopathy is simplified because the remedies are *specific* for certain situations and there are few differentiating characteristics between the remedies which need to be considered.

READING ASSIGNMENT

Read pp. 80-81 in the TEXT, stopping at Obstruction to Breathing.

WRITTEN ASSIGNMENT

13. A woman in her third month of pregnancy is involved in an automobile accident in which her abdomen made contact with the steering wheel. As a result of the trauma she is in a state of partial shock and is bleeding moderately from the uterus. On her way to the hospital, what remedy may be best to give her first? What may be a good choice for the second remedy for her to take? Why?

READING ASSIGNMENT

In the TEXT read pp. 81-84, Obstruction to Breathing, stopping at Shock.

WRITTEN ASSIGNMENT

14. For the drowning victim, along with immediate first aid measures such as mouth-to-mouth resuscitation and cardiopulmonary resuscitation, if necessary, what remedy should be given as soon as possible? What is the best way of administering a homeopathic medicine to an unconscious person?

15. What remedy might a homeopath think to give a child who has developed an asthma attack just after midnight, who feels better from sitting up but feels like suffocating while lying down? The child is restless in bed and has anxiety about health. Find this remedy in the TEXT materia medica and read it. What are the modalities of this remedy?

READING ASSIGNMENT

Read pp. 84-89 in the TEXT.

As we cover more complaints, we find the same homeopathic medicines being used. The characteristics of a remedy usually remain the same no matter what the complaint is.[1]

The Arsenicum fever is similar to the Arsenicum asthma attack in that the suffering subject, in both cases, is anxious, restless, and relieved by warmth.

The Bryonia fever wants to lie very still and is worse from the least movement. This matches the Bryonia joint injury (p. 54 TEXT), which is worse from the least movement. And also the Bryonia broken rib. Imagine having a broken rib; moving would be the last thing you would want to do.

---

1 This phenomenon has been covered in greater depth on p. 22 of this Syllabus.

The Belladonna fever is characterized by having a sudden onset - as a rule the symptoms do not develop gradually over a few days. The person usually has a hot flushed face and the temperature is high. There is often a throbbing pulse and the pupils are dilated. These are the same symptoms as found in the Belladonna sunstroke (p. 90 TEXT).

READING ASSIGNMENT

Read pp. 90-93 in the TEXT.

---

* * * STOP * * *

Before you continue with the next lesson, send to your instructor your responses to all of the written assignments from lessons 1 and 2. If you have any questions about the material covered, send them in to your instructor with your assignments. The address for mailing in your written assignments is given on p. 2 of this Syllabus.

Notes:

LESSON 3

READING ASSIGNMENT

Arsenicum album Materia Medica.
Read Arsenicum album in the TEXT materia medica on p. 259 and, if available, in your remedy kit brochure. Read Arsenicum album in BOERICKE on pp. 79-83, scanning the material by placing emphasis on finding the same symptoms in the TEXT. Read the modalities carefully.

WRITTEN ASSIGNMENT

Arsenicum album Materia Medica
1. *List the outstanding psychological symptoms of Arsenicum.*

2. *Describe the way the Arsenicum person likes to drink.*

3. *Drinks at what temperature improve Arsenicum?*

4. *Name the type of pains for which Arsenicum is famous.*

5. *What temperature generally relieves Arsenicum?*

6. *At what hour or span of time does Arsenicum feel worse?*

7. *What temperature generally makes the Arsenicum state feel worse?*

8. *Write the abbreviation for Arsenicum.*

READING ASSIGNMENT

Belladonna Materia Medica.
Read Belladonna in the TEXT materia medica p. 259 and, if available, in your remedy kit brochure. Read Belladonna in BOERICKE on pp. 110-115, scanning the material by placing emphasis on finding the same symptoms in the TEXT. Read the modalities carefully.

WRITTEN ASSIGNMENT

Belladonna Materia Medica
9. *Choose the words which best describe a Belladonna state from the following selection: gradual, sudden, intense, mild, pale, red.*

10. *What word(s) best describe(s) Belladonna pains?*

11. *How do being exposed to noise, light, and being touched affect the Belladonna state?*

12. *Write the abbreviation for Belladonna.*

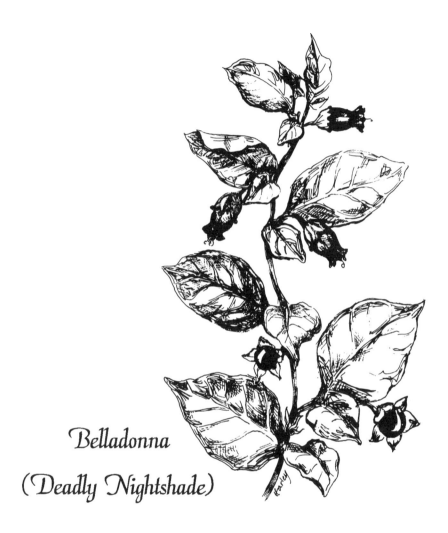

Belladonna

(Deadly Nightshade)

We have begun our practical use of homeopathy with accidents, injuries, and emergencies. Now we need to learn the fundamentals necessary for effective handling of other types of complaints. As we learn Casetaking and Case Analysis, we will be able to utilize these skills for handling a large spectrum of complaints.

In order to put homeopathy into practice we need to become excellent observers. We must become like detectives who carefully observe and record all of the symptoms and characteristics of the ailing person. This process is known as *Casetaking*.

Casetaking

Casetaking is a science and an art, for although it requires a skilled precision, it draws upon our perceptive abilities. In our dialogue with the sick person we must elicit the symptoms of the complaint, through allowing the person to express his suffering in his own words. And we employ a conscious method of questioning the person. While this process is going on, we are at the same time noticing and observing the person's appearance, mood, and other objective signs. During the process of casetaking we need to write down the information received. This constitutes the process of taking the case. It has been said that a case well taken is half of the process leading to selection of a correct remedy. A well taken case makes the process of case analysis and deciding on the remedy much easier. On the other hand, a poorly taken case is difficult to analyze.

Recording the Symptoms

While recording the symptoms, a method is employed for noting the importance or strength of a symptom. Some symptoms will be intense, clear, and readily apparent. Naturally these symptoms will be of greater value for our case analysis. Other symptoms may seem vague or uncertain; obviously we will give these less consideration. The system of underlining the symptoms helps us to note their value.

The general guidelines to follow for the use of underlines is as follows:

No underlines:
> These are symptoms which are vague. The sick person may be unsure about them and would not offer the information without our questioning them.

1 underline:
> These are symptoms which are clear and more definite. They have some intensity, but still we received information about the symptom only after we questioned about it.[2]

2 underlines:
> These are symptoms which are clear and more intense than 1 underline. Here the information about the symptom is volunteered without our having to ask.

3 underlines:
> These are the most clear and intense symptoms which the sick person tells us about without our needing to question. Also, those objective things we directly observe about the patient's appearance and mood, *when obvious*, are considered 3 underlines.[1]

WRITTEN ASSIGNMENT

A homeopath is taking the case of a young woman with a fever:

13. He clearly observes that her skin is red, hot, and dry; and her pupils are dilated. These symptoms would qualify for how many underlines? Why?

---

1 The basis of this schema of underlines has been drawn from George Vithoulkas, *The Science of Homeopathy* (New York: Grove Press, 1980), p. 182.

2 Note that in some cases it is possible to elicit a strong symptom with questioning, that warrants receiving 2 or even 3 underlines.

14. *The first thing she tells him is that her head is throbbing. This symptom would qualify for how many underlines? Why?*

15. *He asks her if any conditions alleviated the throbbing or made it worse. She says that it feels better when she is sitting up. This symptom would qualify for how many underlines? Why?*

16. *He asks her if any condition makes her throbbing pain worse. She cannot think of any. He gives her a multiple choice question, telling many types of modalities which can make pains worse. Finally she answers that she thinks it is a little worse when lying down. This symptom would qualify for how many underlines? Why?*

17. *She tells him that her eyes seem somewhat more sensitive to light than usual. This symptom would qualify for how many underlines? Why?*

By underlining the symptoms while they are still a fresh impression, we will have less to remember. This helps to keep the process of case analysis simplified. In this course, for the sake of simplicity, we will be using the numerals (3), (2), and (1) to indicate the number of underlines. Some homeopaths prefer to place the underlines underneath symptoms or to the left of them. This way is also fine.

Example:

(3) < cold wet weather could also be	< cold wet weather or	☰< cold wet weather
(2) burning pain in stomach	burning pain in stomach	=burning pain in stomach
(1) rawness in throat	rawness in throat	− rawness in throat

READING ASSIGNMENT

Aconite Materia Medica.
Read Aconite in the TEXT materia medica on p. 256 and, if available, in your remedy kit brochure. Read Aconite in BOERICKE on pp. 7-11, scanning the material by placing emphasis on finding the same symptoms in the TEXT. Read the modalities carefully.

WRITTEN ASSIGNMENT

Aconite Materia Medica

18. *Describe the psychological state that typifies Aconite.*

19. *What weather conditions can be an etiology (causation)[1] of an Aconite state?*

1A complete description of Etiology is given on p. 36 of this Syllabus.

20. Describe the onset of Aconite.

21. Describe the thirst of an Aconite patient.

22. Write the abbreviation for Aconite.

When we write down the symptoms it is a good idea to have a separate line for each symptom, with some space underneath it to add the details of the modalities during our necessary questioning.

In our recording of symptoms and subsequent organization of case data which follows in the course work, the general idea is that symptoms which have more underlines get listed first. So a 3 underlined symptom would get listed first, 2 underlined would be next in descending order, and the 0 underlined would naturally be listed last.

For example:
A sick person has nausea and vomiting(3) as soon as cold drinks turn warm in his stomach(2). However, cold drinks temporarily relieve the condition(1). He has a burning pain in the stomach(2), which is better from cold drinks(2). He has fever with chills(1), which seems better from sleep(1) and open air.[1]

> (3) nausea and vomiting
>> (2) as soon as cold drinks turn warm in stomach
>> (1) > cold drinks, temporarily
>
> (2) burning pain in stomach
>> (2) > cold drinks
>
> (1) fever with chills
>> (1) > sleep
>> > open air

Observe how these symptoms have been recorded in descending order of intensity. Note how **nausea and vomiting**, having 3 underlines, is listed first. Likewise notice how the modalities relating to this symptom are listed with the 2 underlined modality coming up first and the one underlined modality listed second. And see that **fever with chills**, the symptom with the least underlines, is listed last.

Notice also how the modalities are indented beneath the symptoms to which they correspond. For example:

> (1) burning pain in the stomach
>> (2) > cold drinks

The modality > cold drinks is indented beneath burning pain in the stomach. It provides visual acuity in showing that the burning stomach pains *are* > cold drinks.

---

1 The remedy best matching these symptoms is Phosphorus/Phos.

WRITTEN ASSIGNMENT

Organize the following cases and rewrite the symptoms and modalities according to the example given above. Use the symbols < >, and indent the modalities beneath the symptoms to which they correspond.

23. Case 1[1]

    A man has sore aching pains in the lower back(3) which feel worse in cold wet weather(3) and from bending(2). He gets relief from hot baths and gets relief from walking(1).

24. Case 2[2]

    A child is stung by a bee. She has burning(2), stinging(2) pains which are aggravated by heat(2). She also has a headache that is worse in the sun(1).

Casetaking - Questioning

Someone may have complained of a pulsating headache. Having recorded this we now need to know what alleviates the pain and/or what aggravates it. Or...

The person may have complained of the headache but has not been able to tell us clearly what the pain feels like.

Here we must employ *conscious questioning.* The main issue in our questioning is that we have to *avoid suggesting an answer.* The question needs to be stated in an *open-ended* manner. For example:

We may ask, "What does the pain feel like?"

Or, assuming we know what a headache feels like (pulsating, for instance), but need to know its modalities, we may ask, "are there any conditions that make the pulsating head pain better or worse?"

Should the person be unable to answer, an open-ended kind of multiple choice question could be posed, such as this:

"There are many types of head pain. If any of these match or are quite close to your pain, let me know." Then we run through a list of many types of pain, such as - pulsating, sore, dull, burning, cutting, sharp, etc. Such a question often helps the person to verbalize the pain accurately. This method could be especially useful in the case of a 7-year-old child who does not have a vocabulary of pain words in the forefront of his or her awareness. Providing the multiple choice question can enable the sufferer to remember a valuable modality or express a pain in his or her own words.

---

1 The remedy best matching these symptoms is Rhus toxicodendron/Rhus tox.
2 The remedy best matching these symptoms is Apis mellifica/Apis.

What type of questioning must we try to *avoid*? The questions which suggest an answer, or require a yes/no answer.

Examples of questioning modes to *avoid*:

Does your headache have a burning pain?

Is your headache better from lying down?

WRITTEN ASSIGNMENT

25. A young 8-year-old earache victim is unable to describe how the pain feels except that "it hurts real bad." Write out a sample of questioning which might be employed to find out the type of pain the child is feeling.

Observation

Those symptoms and conditions which we can notice directly are of particular value. These symptoms are not an interpretation made by the sufferer. These are symptoms and conditions which we can observe are a direct expression of them. This type of observation is especially important in treating those who cannot speak well. Falling into this category would be infants, young children, and those whose illness hampers their ability to articulate. This also applies, of course, when using homeopathy for pets. In these cases it is also valuable to speak with relatives or friends who, having been around to help for a longer period of time, may have noticed some valuable things. These are kinds of things we can observe:

Body temperature reactions, such as whether the sufferer is bundled up and chilly, or if he wants the windows open or closed.

Appearance - such things as the color of the skin, face, and tongue.

How the skin feels - whether it is dry, clammy, cold, hot, etc.

Any odors coming from the subject.

The mood and facial expression - whether it is irritable, timid, crying, or anxious, etc.

Reaction to external stimuli - such things as whether bright light is tolerated, or the need for window shades to be drawn, and the reaction to being touched, and to noise.

The body position - whether lying down, sitting, standing, quiet, or restless.

WRITTEN ASSIGNMENT

26. My neighbor's pet collie has developed an itching skin condition. How can I tell it is itching? - Because I observe her intensely rubbing the area against a rough edged piece of wood. In order to accurately find the correct remedy for her, we need to know how temperature - cold or heat - would affect the itching. Think about it and offer some ideas as to how we could find out these modalities.

KINDS OF INFORMATION TO LOOK FOR IN CASETAKING

Having viewed this process of casetaking, we now examine all of the important symptoms and factors *to look for* in casetaking. Familiarizing ourselves with the kinds of information to elicit makes us more skilled when taking an actual case. Naturally, every situation will vary, and in any given illness we could not expect to elicit all of the symptoms given in this outline. Initially we will not be employing the use of all of these symptoms at once. As we proceed through different types of complaints we will see more and more of these symptoms coming into play. Gradually we will become more familiar with them as we take cases on our own. You should make it a point to refer to this material frequently while casetaking. If you wish to become skillful with homeopathy, it is essential that you become well acquainted with this material. For your easy reference, **The Kinds of Information to Look for in Casetaking** has been reproduced on the back inside cover of this Syllabus.

Cause - Etiology Of The Illness

Were any conditions responsible for the development of the illness? For example, did the illness occur because of exposure to cold wet weather, from exposure to cold dry wind, from over-exposure to the sun, or from dietary indiscretions? These kinds of symptoms, *if* they are present in a case, can lead us quickly to the correct remedy. Note that in order for a condition or situation to be able to qualify as an etiology it has to appear pronounced as clearly the cause of the illness. To be worth noting, an etiology has to be strong. Also, etiology can be especially helpful in the treatment of accidents and injuries - such as over-exertion, a fall on the tailbone, automobile whiplash, etc. In these cases the etiology helps to define the specific injury.

Onset

An illness which appears quickly and with intensity is known as having a sudden onset. An illness which develops gradually is considered to have a slow onset. Onset can be a valuable symptom to look for in some cases. It must be prominent, however, in order for it to be worth taking note of - to have value in case analysis. Also, some complaints have stages where the symptoms change. For example, a cold. The symptoms in the early stages - the onset - of the cold may be different from the cold after it fully develops. In this situation the onset of the cold would be a valuable symptom to make note of in the early stages of the complaint but not for the later stages of the complaint. Further explanation of this is given on p. 50 of this Syllabus, under Focusing on the Symptoms in the Present Moment in Time.

Local Symptoms

LOCATION OF SYMPTOMS
The location of the pain or other discomfort or symptom. Be attentive to notice the precise location of the pain or symptom. In some cases the symptom is only on one side - note that. For example, a right-sided sore throat is characteristic of Belladonna.

SENSATIONS
The sensations of the pain and discomfort. Some examples of common painful sensations are these: aching, sore, pulsating, burning, itching, cutting, bursting, shooting, cramping, pressing, and stitching. Note that the definition of a *stitching* pain is - as if provoked by a point.

DISCHARGES
Note the color, consistency, and odor, if any. Most commonly this is mucus from the nose, throat, and lungs. However, discharges could come from the ears, the skin, or any orifice of the body.

MODALITIES

Modalities are any conditions which make the symptoms better or worse. Some of the more outstanding modalities are:

Modalities of Reaction to Temperature and Weather, such as warm rooms, cold weather, open air, drafts, warm application, cold application, exposure to the sun, and wet or dry weather.

Modalities of Time, such as the hour of day or night; or the more general categories of morning, afternoon, evening, before or after midnight.

Modalities of Rest or Motion. Is the person better or worse from movement or rest?

Modalities of Position of the Body. In some situations the person is worse from lying down; in other situations the person is better standing up. Some cases are improved by lying on the painful side, while others are made worse from doing so.

Modalities of the Effects of Eating or Drinking, such as cold drinks, warm drinks, eating.

Modalities of Reaction to Stimuli, such as the effects of light, noise, conversation, touch: light or firm, massage, clothing touching the affected area.

General Symptoms

General Symptoms are an expression of the 'overall' general body characteristics which are prominent. The most important General Symptoms to look for in casetaking for minor ailments are as follows:

Body temperature - Is the person chilly or warm?
General energy of the person - restless, dull, weak, etc.
The degree of thirst or thirstlessness.
Specific foods or drinks which are craved or detested during the illness.
Perspiration - when and where it occurs; its odor, if any.

General Symptoms are also considered to be any modalities which repeat themselves prominently in a case. For example, consider a child having an earache together with congested nose and cough. The earache, stuffed nose, and cough are *all* made worse from exposure to cold air. The modality of 'worse cold air' would then be considered as a General Symptom.

The Mental / Emotional State (abbreviated as M / E)

The main thing to observe in the personality during an acute illness or injury is the mood as it departs from the normal state. For example, an infant who has been mild and sweet in nature begins to teethe. While teething, the child becomes quite irritable. This irritability, found in the remedy Chamomilla, is a good symptom to emphasize, because normally the child is sweet. Another example would be the child who is independent who, during an illness, has become dependent, with fears of being alone, which is characteristic of Pulsatilla. This child's dependent behavior would be a good symptom to record and emphasize for treating the child's acute illness.[1]

In some cases you will find that the Mental/Emotional state during an acute illness is not much different from the personality when well. For example, a child who is normally dependent and weepy is even more dependent and weepy during a cold. In this case the characteristic of being dependent and weepy *would* be recorded simply because it stands out clearly as a mental/emotional trait which the organism is displaying.

---

1 The analysis of Chronic complaints of long standing requires an advanced training in homeopathy, which goes beyond the scope of this introductory course. With chronic complaints, much more emphasis is placed upon the ongoing Mental/Emotional state of a person. The mental and emotional levels represent deeper expressions of health in the Hierarchy of Health, as explained in this Syllabus, Lesson 1, p. 11.

WRITTEN ASSIGNMENT

27. From the outline we have just read of all of the symptoms and factors to look for in casetaking, list the outline headings that are given. Be sure to include each of the six modalities. Note: **The Kinds of Information to Look for in Casetaking** *is an essential component in your study and application of homeopathy. Return to it often.*

READING ASSIGNMENT

Pulsatilla Materia Medica.
Read Pulsatilla in the TEXT materia medica on p. 268 and, if available, in your remedy kit brochure. Read Pulsatilla in BOERICKE on pp. 536-539, scanning the material by placing emphasis on finding the same symptoms in the TEXT. Read the modalities carefully.

Note: Add this one important symptom for Pulsatilla. The mucus is *easily expectorated:* it comes out easily.

WRITTEN ASSIGNMENT

Pulsatilla Materia Medica
28. Describe the temperament of Pulsatilla.
29. Describe the classic Pulsatilla discharge.
30. What temperature aggravates the Pulsatilla complaint?
31. What environmental factors improve a Pulsatilla complaint?
32. Write the abbreviation for Pulsatilla.

Format For Recording The Symptoms

Examine now the following case of Influenza, with the case written out in a narration and an organized format. The narration is merely intended to simulate the mass of symptoms from a casetaking interview. Our goal in recording symptoms is to intelligently organize them. Therefore try to organize your case data along the lines of the organized format given below. This format is designed to facilitate case analysis for minor acute complaints.

Note: Remember the number in ( ) parentheses following each symptom is the number of underlines for that symptom.

NARRATION:

Influenza in a girl twelve years old: The symptoms developed gradually (3) over a period of a week during the hottest week of the summer (2). Her expression is dull and weak (3). She has an intensely sore throat (3), with red, inflamed tonsils (3). Swallowing is difficult (2) and causes a shooting pain from the throat to the ears (2). She has a dull headache (2) which is better from moving around (1), better from cool open air, and worse from damp weather (2). All of her throat pains are worse from damp weather (2). She has a dry cough (1), which is worse from damp weather (2). She has a low fever with chills down her back (2) and a yellow coated tongue (2). Her discernings appear to be lethargied (3). In the interview she was slow to respond and answer questions.[1]

---

[1] The symptoms in this case are characteristic of the remedy, Gelsemium / Gels.

ORGANIZED FORMAT

CHIEF COMPLAINT - Influenza
ETIOLOGY - (2) exposure to hot weather
ONSET - (3) gradual

LOCAL SYMPTOMS
    Sore Throat
        (3) Sore pain in throat
            (2)< damp weather
        (3) Tonsils red and inflamed
        (2) Shooting pain from throat to ears on swallowing.
            (2)< damp weather
        (2) Swallowing difficult
        (2) Dull Headache
            (2) < damp weather
            (1) > movement
              > cool open air
        (2) Fever with chills
        (2) Tongue coated yellow
        (1) Cough, Dry
            (2) < damp weather

GENERAL SYMPTOMS
    (3) Dull, weak
        (2) < damp weather

MENTAL / EMOTIONAL STATE (M/E)
    (3) Lethargic
    Answers slowly

Notice how the bulk of the symptoms has been classified into three Main categories; **Local Symptoms, General Symptoms, and the Mental/Emotional State.** Refer back to the outline on pp. 36-37 Syllabus at this time so that you have a sound understanding of what constitutes the Local Symptoms, General Symptoms, and the Mental/Emotional State. Once we take a case we need to organize our case data into these basic categories.

Notice how within each category the symptoms are listed in the sequence of the number of underlines in descending order of intensity. Find the Dull Headache in the above example, with the corresponding Modalities beneath it. Notice how the Modalities are also listed in this descending order of intensity.

Note how the Modality of worse damp weather repeats itself. The sore throat, and headache and the cough all worse from damp weather. When a Modality is clear and it repeats itself in a case, it becomes a General Symptom. Refer back to p. 37 Syllabus and review this explanation in General Symptoms.

Note in the above sample format how the Modality of being better cool open air, is not considered a General Symptom. In this case only the headache is better from cool open air. In order for a Modality to be considered also as a General Symptom, it needs to 'run through' the case. It needs to also be present relating to other symptoms so that one is enabled to conclude that the Modality is an expression of the 'general overall' state.

This format for recording symptoms is intended to serve as an example to provide a framework for recording the cases you take. To illustrate this format, we have used a hypothetical example in this case of influenza. Keep in mind however, that in any given acute case, one doesn't always find an Etiology, Onset or even Mental/Emotional symptoms pronounced enough to be worth recording.

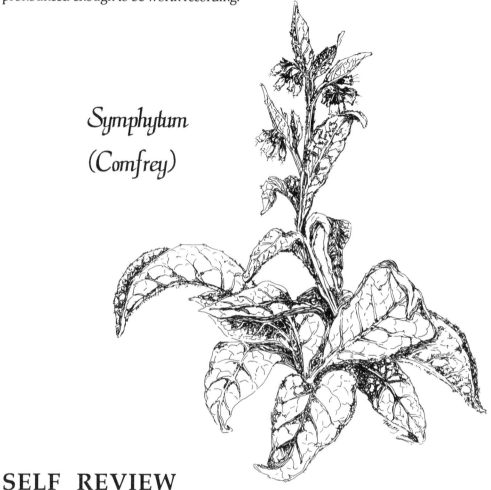

Symphytum

(Comfrey)

SELF REVIEW

Affirm the material presented thus far by completing the following multiple choice questions. The answers are on p. 43 of this Syllabus. Should you have any questions, write them down and send them in to your instructor together with the written assignments for Lessons 3 and 4.

1. Examine the following list of case data:

    Pulsating pain over the left eye; > warm applications
    Bleeding gums
    Rattling cough at night
    Itching eyes; < rubbing

    How may the above case data be best classified? (choose one)

    A. General Symptoms
    B. Etiology
    C. Local Symptoms
    D. All of the above
    E. Mental/Emotional Symptoms

2. Which of the following formats is most accurately organized?[1]

A.
CHIEF COMPLAINT - Sore throat
ETIOLOGY - (3) Drafts of cold air
ONSET - (3) Sudden
LOCAL SYMPTOMS
    (3) Constricting sensation right side of throat
        (3)   < swallowing
        (2)   < while speaking
              < drinking liquids
        (3) thirstless
        (2) constant desire to swallow

GENERAL SYMPTOMS
    (3) Flushed face
    (1) Restless

MENTAL/EMOTIONAL SYMPTOMS
    (1) Irritable

B.
CHIEF COMPLAINT - Sore throat
ETIOLOGY - (3) Drafts of cold air
ONSET - (3) Sudden
LOCAL SYMPTOMS
    (3) Constricting sensation right side of throat
        (3)   < swallowing
        (2)   < while speaking
              < drinking liquids
    (2) Constant desire to swallow

GENERAL SYMPTOMS
    (3) Flushed face
    (3) Thirstless
    (1) Restless
    (1) Irritable

C.
CHIEF COMPLAINT - Sore throat
ETIOLOGY - Drafts of cold air
ONSET - (3) Sudden
LOCAL SYMPTOMS
    (3) Constricting sensation right side of throat
        (3   < swallowing
        (2)   < while speaking
              < drinking liquids
    (2) Constant desire to swallow

GENERAL SYMPTOMS
    (3) Flushed face
    (3) Thirstless
    (1) Restless

MENTAL/EMOTIONAL SYMPTOMS
    (1) Irritable

D.
CHIEF COMPLAINT - Sore throat
ETIOLOGY - (3) Drafts of cold air
ONSET - (3) Sudden
LOCAL SYMPTOMS
    (3) Constricting sensation right side of throat
        (2)   < while speaking
        (3)   < swallowing
              < drinking liquids
    (2) Constant desire to swallow

GENERAL SYMPTOMS
    (3) Flushed face
    (3) Thirstless
    (1) Restless

MENTAL/EMOTIONAL SYMPTOMS
    Irritable

---

1 The symptoms presented in this question are characteristic of the remedy, Belladonna/Bell.

3. Which of the following formats is most accurately organized?[1]

A.
CHIEF COMPLAINT - Earache
LOCAL SYMPTOMS
    (3) Throbbing pain in ears
        (2)   < warmth
        (1)   > open air
    (1) Congested nose, yellow mucus
        (3) < warmth
        (1) > open air
        (1) < evening
GENERAL SYMPTOMS
    (2) < warmth
    (1) > open air
    (1) thirstless
MENTAL/EMOTIONAL SYMPTOMS
    (3) Cries easily
    (2) Desires company

B.
CHIEF COMPLAINT - Earache
LOCAL SYMPTOMS
    (3) Throbbing pains in ears
        (2) < warmth
        (1) > open air
    (1) Congested nose, yellow mucus
        (2) < warmth
        (1) > open air
        (1) < evening
GENERAL SYMPTOMS
    (1) Thirstless
MENTAL/EMOTIONAL SYMPTOMS
    (3) Cries easily
    (2) Desires company

C.
CHIEF COMPLAINT - Earache
LOCAL SYMPTOMS
    (3) Throbbing pains in ears
        (2) < warmth
        (1) > open air
    (1) Congested nose, yellow mucus
        (2) < warmth
        (1) > open air
        (1) < evening
GENERAL SYMPTOMS
    (1) Thirstless
MENTAL/EMOTIONAL SYMPTOMS
    (2) Desires company
    (3) Cries easily

D.
CHIEF COMPLAINT - Earache
LOCAL SYMPTOMS
    (1) Congested nose, yellow mucus
        (2) < warmth
        (1) > open air
        (1) < evening
    (3) Throbbing pains in ears
        (2) < warmth
        (1) > open air
GENERAL SYMPTOMS
    (2) < warmth
    (1) > open air
    (1) Thirstless
MENTAL/EMOTIONAL SYMPTOMS
    (3) Cries easily
    (2) Desires company

---

1 The symptoms presented in this question are characteristic of the remedy, Pulsatilla/Puls.

WRITTEN ASSIGNMENT

33. Now it is time for you to take a case of an acute illness. Note that an acute illness is a complaint of temporary duration usually of less than 3 weeks time, which can be treated at home using self-care. So find someone with an acute ailment, it could be a family member, a friend or anyone. The case you choose to take could be something simple like an injury, indigestion, an earache, congested nose, sore throat or any one of the scores of ailments mentioned in the TEXT. You should have NO DIFFICULTY in finding someone with one of these ailments. It is very likely that the ailment you will choose will not have as many symptoms and multiple ailments as the example on p. 39 Syllabus, that is fine. You are advised to actively seek to take the case of an acute illness at this time, without delay.

Keep in front of you the outline on back cover of this Syllabus of the possible **Kinds of Information to Look for in Casetaking.** *Each ailment and individual case is unique, do not expect to elicit ALL the information given in the outline for each case you take. While casetaking your powers of observation will be exercised as you learn to become fluent with the method of questioning. Do not worry as yet about analyzing the case. Concentrate on taking it well. After recording the information, go back and rewrite it in a format like the one given on p. 39 Syllabus. Use a fresh sheet of paper. Try to get all the symptoms in an organized format on one side of a sheet whenever possible. By recording the symptoms closer to the left hand margin of the paper, you will have more room for doing the case analysis work which is in the following lessons. Eventually with experience you will be able to record the symptoms in the organized format during casetaking, without having to rewrite them.*

Send this one case, in an organized format, in as written assignment # 33. It is recommended that you get practical experience by taking numerous cases, but only send one in to your instructor, upon completing Lesson 4.

Do not send in your narration or first draft of the symptoms, unless of course they do not require revision and already are in a well organized format.

Casetaking Hint

You will be more effective in your casetaking as a beginner if you follow this advice: Prior to taking the case, find out (if you can), what the main (chief) complaint is. Then refer in the TEXT to the remedy descriptions relating to that complaint and read through them.

This serves to refresh your memory and activate your mind so that you will recognize the most important symptoms. It is a good idea to have the TEXT open to the complaint when taking the case. By referring to it, you may be reminded to observe something or ask a question you otherwise would not have considered. Remember, however, to keep your questions open ended.

SELF REVIEW ANSWERS:
3. A
2. C
1. C

LESSON 4

Case Analysis I

There is a series of common-sense moves that go through the mind of a skilled homeopath during case analysis. These appear automatic to the experienced homeopath. Most texts do not attempt to instruct us in the intricacies of these common-sense decisions. They assume that by providing a framework, the motived beginner will in time find his/her own way and pick up the *art* of these skills. In this course we learn the basics of these skills.

Let us follow these processes of analysis together. The written assignments are an opportunity to give you practice and clarify any points of ambiguity. Initially the early case analysis assignments will be more obvious cases, getting you accustomed to the procedures. Later we will solve less obvious cases. After you become somewhat fluent with these thought processes through experience, they will become a common-sense second-nature aspect of your case analysis.

Case analysis is a learning-by-doing experience. Experienced homeopaths have elaborate methods of case analysis, using texts which list the symptoms in great detail, known as repertories. Time-saving versions of these repertories have recently been developed for computer use. In this introductory course we will be referring to the simplified descriptions for each complaint in the TEXT. And we will seek to find the description that best matches the complaint. If the information is not complete enough in the chart or specific chapter in the TEXT, we will be referring to the TEXT materia medica, or finally to BOERICKE to those remedies which look close so that we may choose the one remedy that matches best.

We have taken a case and have recorded the symptoms which have been graded with our system of underlines. The recorded information has been placed into an organized format. The remedy we choose will be based upon this information.

When analyzing our case data we look in the appropriate chapter(s) of the TEXT to find the one remedy that best matches all the symptoms. This process of matching the remedy to the symptoms is accomplished by recording the abbreviations of the homeopathic remedies next to symptoms to which they correspond. The following example illustrates this:

CHIEF COMPLAINT - Fever

GENERAL SYMPTOMS
>   (3) Restlessness   ACON. ARS. BELL.
>   (2) Thirst for large quantities of water   ACON. BRY. PHOS.
>   (2) One cheek red, the other pale   ACON. CHAM.
>   (1) Hot dry skin   ACON. BELL.

While looking up the fever remedies in the TEXT descriptions on p. 89, examining the TEXT charts on pp. 94 - 101 for the fever remedies, and looking to the TEXT materia medica for more details, we place the remedy abbreviations next to the symptoms they match. So after all the symptoms are matched we can then visually count up which of the remedies match our symptom data most thoroughly. This method keeps us from having to use all of the findings from our memory. In this case, Aconite best covers the symptoms.

Note, in the above case, that no Onset has been recorded. Aconite, and Belladonna are famous for having rapid intense onsets. So in this case, when seeing the remedy Aconite figuring prominently we could make an additional inquiry to see if the onset is rapid, had we neglected to do so earlier while taking the case. That would serve as a further confirmation that Aconite is the remedy. It is common for homeopaths to ask of their clients additional confirming and differentiating questions while they are hot on the trail of the curative remedy.

In the above Fever case, the strongest symptom is the (3) Restlessness. The correct remedy in any given case will, almost always, be one of the remedies that corresponds to the strongest symptom(s) of the Chief Complaint. In this case (3) Restlessness is the strongest symptom of the Fever. We would tend to conclude that the correct remedy would most likely be one of the main remedies which has Fever with restlessness: ACON. ARS. or BELL. Therefore, try to be as thorough as possible when searching for remedies that correspond to the most prominent symptoms in a case.

We see that the symptom (2) Thirst for large quantities of water during fever corresponds to ACON. BRY. PHOS. Note that ACON. appears again. BRY. appears for the first time. Could BRY. be the correct remedy? Probably not in this case; BRY. does not have restlessness, BRY. wants to be very still. PHOS. is another remedy which has intense thirst, yet it does not have the pronounced restlessness during fever. Why then is it necessary to record the remedies BRY. and PHOS. at all? Well, if you are totally sure of yourself and you are sure that the restlessness during fever is a very strong symptom, then it is not absolutely necessary to record the remedies which do not apply. It is safer, however, for the beginner to record all the remedies that match this symptom, because it is 2 underlines and there are so few symptoms in this case.

Note that the symptom (1) Hot dry skin during fever has ACON. and BELL. which are two remedies that have been recorded in the first most important symptom of the case. If, however, the hot dry skin during fever had many other remedies which *did not* correspond to the more important symptoms in the case, *then* we could leave out matching those extraneous remedies.

Note that in this Fever case all of the symptoms are General Symptoms. Most of the time a case will also have Local Symptoms with Modalities. However it should be remembered that each case is unique unto itself. Refer back to p. 37 in this Syllabus to review the definition of General Symptoms if you are unclear on this.

The search to find the remedies which match the symptoms needs to be made with careful thoroughness. In this introductory stage of homeopathy for minor ailments, the TEXT is our major reference source. For each of the ailments covered, the TEXT lists the outstanding remedies to be considered, with their keynote characteristics as they apply to that ailment. This Syllabus also contains supplementary remedy differentials on common ailments which are locateable through the Syllabus Index.

Cultivate the habit of searching carefully for the remedies corresponding to the symptoms. In doing so you will be receiving the benefits of becoming thoroughly familiar with your homeopathic reference books, which will make you more adept each time they are used. Another benefit which we derive from this work is that we become more familiar with the keynotes of the homeopathic remedies by repeatedly seeing the symptoms to which they correspond.

READING ASSIGNMENT

Read the Sore Throat Differential that follows in the Syllabus. This material is supplementary to the TEXT.

Sore Throat Differential

The main factors to consider include onset, degree of thirst, which side of the throat is affected, sensations on swallowing, appearance of throat, effects of warm or cold drinks.

Belladonna / Bell.
A common remedy for superficial sore throat. The onset is sudden and there may be an intense fever. The throat is red and dry and the glands of the neck are swollen. The face is flushed and pupils are dilated. The pains are burning or throbbing and it is painful to swallow. More common in right sided sore throats. Usually not thirsty.

Phytolacca / Phyt.
Dark red-bluish throat with swollen tonsils what can have white spots on them. Glands on neck are swollen. Swallowing causes a sharp pain to the right ear. Worse with warm drinks. Can appear restless and frightened. Body feels achy all over.

Arsenicum album / Ars.
Burning pain in throat which is improved by hot drinks. Sore throat worse on right side. Worse after midnight. Restless, can be anxious.

Lycopodium / Lyc.
Burning pain in throat. Better with warm drinks. Starts on right side, then spreads to the left side. Worse 4 - 8 p.m.

Ferrum phos / Ferr p.
Non-descript sore throat; both sides. Given in early stages. Face may be flushed but the person is cool to touch.

Mercurius viv. or sol. / Merc.
Sore throat with offensive breath, and excessive salivation, drools on pillow. Tongue may be puffy. Indented tongue, which means that the outer edge of the tongue has an 'indented' appearance from pressing against the teeth (See illustration on p. 67 Syllabus). Worse at night. Worse from both cold and hot but especially worse from heat of bed.

Hepar sulph / Hep.
Whole throat sensitive, sharp sticking pains in throat. Can come on from exposure to cold dry weather. Glands of neck are very sensitive to touch. Chilly and worse from the cold and better from warmth and warm drinks. Pain may extend to ear. Irritable.

Lachesis / Lach.
Starts on left side and spreads to right side. Intolerant of slightest clothing touching the throat. It is easier to swallow solids or cold liquids. Swallowing hot liquids or empty swallowing is more difficult.

Rhus toxicodendron / Rhus tox.
From over-exertion of vocal cords or exposure to cold wet weather. Hoarseness. Better warm drinks. Achy stiffness, restlessness. Neck can be stiff and achy.

Gelsemium / Gels.
Sore throat with malaise. Very tired, weak. Starts on the left side.

WRITTEN ASSIGNMENT

Read the following case data and give the name of the remedy which best matches each case. Refer to the Syllabus Sore Throat Differential. If wished, you may write the abbreviation of the remedies next to the matching symptoms. Refer the the TEXT materia medica or BOERICKE to confirm your decision and learn more about the remedy.

1. What is the remedy for this sore throat?

LOCAL SYMPTOMS
        (3) < swallowing hot liquids
        (3) < after sleep
        (2) < on left side
        (2) < from clothing and external touch
        (1) tonsils purple

2. What is the remedy for this sore throat?

ETIOLOGY
        (2) Exposure to cold dry weather
LOCAL SYMPTOMS
        (2) Cervical glands (glands of neck) sore
            (2) < touch
        (1) Sticking pains in throat
            (3) > warm drinks
GENERAL SYMPTOMS
        (3) Chilly; sensitive to drafts
M/E
        (1) Irritable

3. What is the remedy for this sore throat?

LOCAL SYMPTOMS
        (2) Burning pain in throat
            (3) > hot drinks
            (2) < 12:30 a.m.
            (1) > head raised up on pillow
M/E
        (1) Anxious

4. What is the remedy for this sore throat?

LOCAL SYMPTOMS
      (3) Throbbing pain right side throat
      (3) Burning pain in throat
          (3) < noise   (Note - these modalities apply to both the
          (3) < sudden movement   throbbing pain and burning pain in throat)
          (1) < liquids
      (3) Throat feels dry

Colds, Flu and Related Conditions

READING ASSIGNMENT

Read now pp. 104 - 110 up to Coughs, in the TEXT.

In using homeopathy for colds and flu, whether dealing with a cold or flu, we must consider all the remedies indicated for both colds and flu. Technically there is a difference between the influenza virus and the cold virus. However, influenza is often preceded by a cold, and the symptoms are often the same for both colds and flu.

The TEXT covers colds and related conditions for Infants in Chapter 8 and Children in Chapter 9. When treating these age groups, we will refer first to these chapters. Then if further clarification is needed we will refer back to Chapter 6 in the TEXT and Syllabus Lesson 4, which goes into more detail on these complaints.

> NOTE: The person who is experiencing chronically recurring colds and related conditions should see an experienced homeopath. Homeopathy can remove the predisposition to these complaints. The TEXT mentions a 'cold and flu tablet'. This 'cold and flu tablet' is the remedy, Influenzinum, which could be given by an experienced homeopath as part of a preventative constitutional treatment program.

Rhus toxicodendron / Rhus tox.
This is an important Flu remedy, which has not been considered for Flu in the TEXT. Incorporate this information into the TEXT's other Flu remedies.

Flu brought on by exposure to cold wet weather.
Flu with aching in the bones, and muscular stiffness.
Sometimes can have a herpetic eruption or cold sore around mouth.
Thick yellow or greenish mucus discharges.
Hoarseness, red scratchy throat, sneezing and coughing.

Improved by warmth.
Improved by movement.
The nose can be more obstructed on the side lain on.

Thirsty for cold drinks.
Restlessness, especially at night.

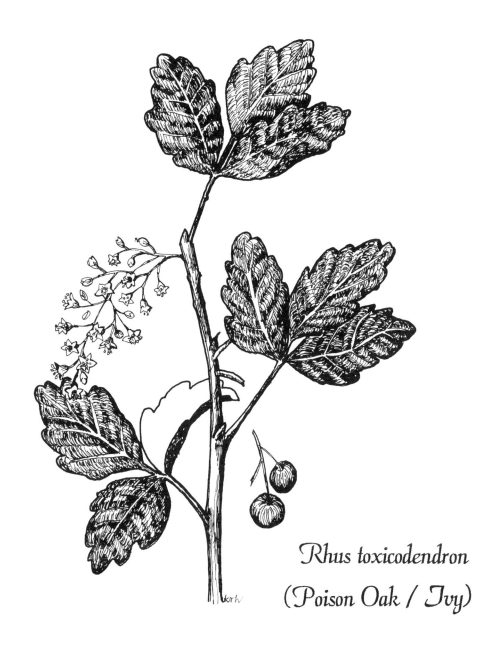

Rhus toxicodendron
(Poison Oak / Ivy)

READING ASSIGNMENT

Eupatorium perfoliatum/Eup. per. is another common Flu remedy. Although it is not in the TEXT materia medica, it is described on p. 109 and in the chart on p. 119. Study the symptoms of this remedy for the Flu on these pages and then turn to p. 274 BOERICKE and read the remedy there, with an emphasis placed on finding symptoms that agree with the description in the TEXT.

Evolution of the Cold and Related Conditions

Colds and their related conditions often have an evolution. There is the period, either rapid or gradual, when they are just beginning to develop: the Onset, the incubation period. And there is the later stage of the ripe cold with all of its symptoms. Some homeopathic remedies are indicated more for Onset and early cold stages. Other remedies are indicated more for the symptoms of a ripe cold.

Focusing on Symptoms in the Present Moment in Time

The rule is to give the remedy which matches the present symptoms. A cold requiring one remedy for the Onset, may require a different remedy at the ripe state. This means that we need to be mobile in homeopathy and open to changing the remedy, when necessary. It would be necessary to change the remedy when the symptoms for which the remedy was given have changed. This can happen when a remedy picture goes from the Onset stage to the ripe stage.

Homeopathy for the Early Stages of Colds and Related Conditions

An advantage of homeopathy is that it is effective in resolving the earliest stages hinting of a cold and the onset of a cold. Approached in this manner, usually the cold never develops. It is aborted; cut short. Or if it does develop, the intensity and duration are much less. The main remedies to consider for the **early stage** of colds are as follows:

Aconite	Anas Barbariae Hepatis Et Cordis
Belladonna	Ferrum phos

Anas Barbariae Hepatis Et Cordis[1] is derived from the heart and liver tissue of a duck, which is high in DNA and RNA. Ducks live in lakes where flu viruses thrive in abundance. It has been found that these flu viruses are harbored within ducks who have been linked to the spread of flu.[2] Anas Barbariae Hepatis et Cordis seems to have a unique capacity in the prevention and resolution of flus, colds and related conditions. Whereas most homeopathic medicines are considered in an individualized manner to match a particular symptom picture, Anas Barbariae Hepatis et Cordis is a general remedy for colds and flu. It does not require an individualized case analysis. This remedy may be taken according to the indication on the product label as a preventative to ward off colds and flu, and during a cold or flu to hasten its resolution.

In situations where there is a syndrome of recurring colds and flu, the Syllabus recommends that you seek deeper constitutional homeopathic treatment under the care of a competent homeopathic physician/practitioner. If Anas Barbariae Hepatis et Cordis needs to be given frequently, it is a sign that this deeper treatment is called for. Remember, the definition of health on the physical plane includes being free from special treatments. That includes the too frequent use of even homeopathic medicines. A homeopathic physician/practitioner can remove the underlying predisposition to the colds and flu. As a result of such treatment your mental, emotional, and physical levels of being will be healthier, more balanced, and ultimately the frequency of these recurring colds and flus will be reduced.

For those persons who are already under the care of a homeopath, it is advisable that they obtain approval from their practitioner before taking Anas Barbariae Hepatis et Cordis on their own. This remedy is commonly available in the 200C potency which is a higher potency remedy and possible interference with a deeper ongoing homeopathic treatment should be avoided.

---

1 This remedy was originally created and researched in Europe by Laboratoires Boiron.
2 Jay Stuller, "Duck/Flu Season, Quack...Quack...Quack-choo!," American Health (December 1987), p.8.

Assessing the Results of the Remedy

It is important to make an effort to really study the well taken symptoms thoroughly to arrive at the best matching remedy. As a rule it is wise to allow at least 12 hours (12 to 24 hours with colds and related conditions) to assess the effect of the cold remedy we have given. In some cases it may be the correct remedy and yet the effect may be evident only after half a day. If we were to become impatient and prematurely give another remedy, we could mistakenly be giving up on the correct remedy. So the rule is to choose carefully and wait *at least 12 hours* before considering a change. How do we assess the progress of a case? We examine the person's suffering and energy. We see he or she is feeling better. When we see the chief symptoms of the complaint begin to subside and the energy improve, we know sufferer is on the road to recovery.

The Interplay Between Case Analysis, Casetaking, and Study of Materia Medica

In practical life situations you may be analyzing the case of a friend or family member which you have just taken. During or at the conclusion of the Case Analysis you may find that more than one remedy seems to match. The way to make the correct remedy selection then lies in looking up these similar remedies in the materia medica - BOERICKE. One scans over those remedies in BOERICKE, looking for other differentiating aspects which can be questioned of or observed in the patient. To illustrate this, assume the following case is one which you have just taken. Follow the commentary and write the abbreviations of the remedies which match the symptoms into this Syllabus. Use a pencil so that corrections can easily be made. Examine the Flu remedies given on pp. 108 - 109 TEXT and those in this Syllabus on pp. 48-49 to facilitate your matching work. Then pick out the two remedies which seem to come closest to matching these symptoms for Flu.

Flu - A Case Analysis Example

Samuel comes down with the Flu. At the Onset he was chilly and very restless and was given Aconite 30C, two doses in one day with slight improvement. The symptom picture then changed after one day to an achy Influenza. Now the symptoms he is currently experiencing are as follows.

> CHIEF COMPLAINT - Influenza
>
> LOCAL SYMPTOMS
>   (3) Aching bones
>   > warmth
>   < movement
>   (2) Achy soreness of eyeballs
>   (1) < movement
>
> GENERAL SYMPTOMS
>   (2) Thirsty

Note: We have not recorded the Onset at this time because the Onset stage has passed. Remember we focus on the symptoms in the present moment in time.

DO NOT PROCEED ONTO THE NEXT PAGE UNTIL YOU HAVE COMPLETED THIS CASE ANALYSIS.

CHIEF COMPLAINT - Influenza

LOCAL SYMPTOMS
         (3) Aching bones ARS. EUP. PER. RHUS TOX.
           > warmth ARS. RHUS TOX.
           < movement EUP. PER.
         (2) Achy soreness of eyeballs EUP. PER.
           < movement EUP. PER.

GENERAL SYMPTOMS
         (2) Thirsty ARS. EUP. PER. RHUS TOX.

The remedies which appear close are EUP. PER. (Eupatorium perfoliatum) and RHUS TOX. (Rhus toxicodendron). The symptoms are in favor of EUP. PER. because of the achy soreness of the eyes, which are made worse by movement.

The situation would have been different if the achiness in the eyes was a vague uncertain symptom, and the modality of worse movement was not present. What would we do in this case if our key symptom clues were taken away? In real life, obtaining symptoms which are clear and accurate is not always easy. In this situation, all remedies - ARS., EUP. PER. and RHUS TOX. would appear to be possibilities. What could we do?

We would need to go to the Materia Medica to read about the remedies in greater detail in order to decide. In this situation we could refer to BOERICKE to examine these remedies. While we are studying BOERICKE it is important to fix in our minds the idea of looking for other characteristic symptoms of the remedy that we have not yet elicited from Samuel, so that we may observe or question him further about them. For example, EUP. PER. is improved by conversation. We may be able to find out if his aching pains are better from talking. The tongue appearance may be helpful, as with RHUS TOX. the tongue can have a red triangular mark at the tip. The EUP. PER. tongue is yellow and coated and the ARS. tongue can be dry, clean and red. The thirst could be important. ARS. is thirsty for sips of warm drinks. RHUS TOX. is thirsty for cold drinks, especially milk.

When casetaking, remember to refer often to the **Kinds of Things to Look for in Casetaking** on p. 36 Syllabus. By taking each case thoroughly, you will have plenty of differentiating symptoms, which, when analyzed, should point to the correct remedy.

Plussing

Plussing is a technique for increasing the potency of a homeopathic remedy. The remedy is dissolved in water and through a process of repeated dilution and stirring of the solution, the potency is increased.

In our use of homeopathy for emergencies, some cases may have really severe pains or symptoms which match a remedy clearly. In this situation we may find that a lower potency remedy such as is found in most home remedy kits provides a definite immediate relief, which, however, is short lived, and the same symptoms soon return. Upon repeating the remedy we notice the same pattern of relief followed by relapse. This is often an indication that the remedy is correct, but the potency is not strong enough to have a decisive effect. Emergencies seem to have a way of happening at inconvenient times, when it may not be possible to gain fast access to a higher potency of the same remedy. In this situation we do have a way out - a course of action developed by the founding father of homeopathy, Samuel Hahnemann. The procedure is known as **Plussing** and it enables us to increase the potency of the homeopathic remedy we have on hand.

The Technique of Plussing

You will need: a clean glass
                      a clean spoon
                      a clean saucer
                      pure water: spring, distilled or filtered

1. Rinse glass, spoon and saucer with pure water to remove any possible surface residues.

2. Fill up glass half-full of pure water and add 3 to 5 pellets or tablets of the needed remedy into it.

3. Stir the water vigorously with spoon for several minutes until the remedy is dissolved.

4. Have the person needing the remedy sip water from the glass until there is some relief. Then stop sipping.

5. Then empty out glass of water, leaving only a few remaining drops clinging to the sides and bottom of glass.

6. Again, fill glass half-full of pure water and stir it vigorously for several minutes. Place the saucer on top of glass to protect it from dust and odor.

7. If/when the symptoms return sip again from glass until there is relief. Then stop sipping.

8. Then repeat steps 5 & 6.

9. If/when the symptoms return sip until there is relief.

10. Repeat steps 5 & 6.

Each time that the glass is emptied, filled and stirred, the potency of the remedy becomes stronger. During this process it is important to keep the glass out of direct sunlight.

The technique of Plussing is useful in some emergencies. Plussing can also be used in any other situation where the remedy is correct but the potency is not strong enough.

* * * STOP * * *

Before you continue with the next lesson, send to your instructor your responses to all of the written assignments from Lessons 3 and 4. If you have any questions about the material covered this far, now is the time to send them in to your instructor with your written assignments.

Notes:

LESSON 5

Case Analysis II

It is essential that one approach case analysis armed with guiding perspectives. You need to be able to view a case in a simplified manner, going first to look for the most important symptoms. Without these guidelines one could easily get bogged down in the process of matching remedies to the symptoms without any overall direction. Unless you have a homeopathic computer program, you will want to avoid matching every remedy which corresponds to every symptom independently of each other. The symptoms in a case are interrelated and we analyze them cleverly, emphasizing the most important ones.

In any given case we can have the following categories:

> Chief Complaint
> Etiology
> Onset
> Local Symptoms
> General Symptoms
> Mental/Emotional Symptoms

Note: Each case is unique and not every case will have each of these categories.

1. As a rule, with acute complaints the first symptoms to which one seeks to match the remedies (analyze), are the strongest symptoms in the case, together with their modalities. Usually these symptoms will have two or three underlines and will be a clear expression of the Chief Complaint. As expressed earlier, it is important that we be especially thorough in finding all the remedies which correspond to these symptoms.

Example: CHIEF COMPLAINT - A Cold [1]
LOCAL SYMPTOMS
(3) Irritating, watery discharge from eyes
(2) < warmth
(1) bland nasal discharge
GENERAL SYMPTOM
(3) Redness of cheeks

In this case, therefore, we first would find the remedies which matched the Local Symptoms:

(3) Irritating watery discharge from eyes
(2) < warmth

2. Next, if the case has a definite Etiology and/or Onset, one then looks to see which of the remedies that corresponded to the strongest Local Symptoms *also* match the Etiology and/or Onset.

---

[1] Note: In this case we would not start by recording every remedy which matches the term - 'A Cold', because it is too non-descript to have any value for our analysis.

Example: CHIEF COMPLAINT - Earache
                      ONSET - (3) sudden
                      LOCAL SYMPTOMS
                          (3) Throbbing pains in chest
                              (2) < heat

We first match the remedies to:
                      (3) Throbbing pain in ears   ACON. BELL. PULS.

Then we match the remedies which have throbbing pains in the ears being worse heat.
                      (2) < heat   ACON. PULS.

So then we have:
                      CHIEF COMPLAINT - Earache
                      ONSET - (3) sudden
                      LOCAL SYMPTOMS
                          (3) Throbbing pain in ears ACON. BELL. PULS.
                              (2) < heat ACON. PULS.

Then we look up the earache remedies which match throbbing pain in ears - ACON. BELL. PULS., to see which has sudden onset.
                      CHIEF COMPLAINT - Earache
                      ONSET - (3) sudden ACON. BELL.
                      LOCAL SYMPTOMS
                          (3) Throbbing pains in ears ACON. BELL. PULS.
                              (2 < heat ACON. PULS.

The Etiology and/or Onset, when clear, will often give you a good clue to the correct remedy. However, many cases do not have a clear etiology or onset. In the above example case ACON. - Aconite is figuring the strongest thus far.

3. Then one looks to analyze other important symptoms in the case. Remember that each case will be different. One looks for -
          A. Strong General Symptom(s)
          Be on the lookout for Modalities in the case which show a pattern of repeating themselves and thus are also considered a General Symptom. This would make a strong General Symptom which the correct remedy would almost have to match.
          B. Strong Mental/Emotional Symptom(s)
          C. Other Local Symptoms

The analysis is further illustrated with this complete case example:
                      CHIEF COMPLAINT - Earache

                      ONSET (3) sudden ACON. BELL.
                      LOCAL SYMPTOMS
                          (3) Throbbing pains in ears ACON. BELL. PULS.
                              (2) < warm room ACON. PULS.
                                    Burning pain in throat ACON. BELL.
                              (2) < warm room ACON.

                      GENERAL SYMPTOMS
                          (3) Thirsty ACON.
                          (2) < warm room ACON.

                      MENTAL/EMOTIONAL SYMPTOMS
                          (2) Restless ACON. BELL.

Symptom (3) Thirsty. It is important in this case. ACON. - Aconite is
)th BELL. - Belladonna and PULS. - Pulsatilla are thirstless as a rule. So
rtant the General Symptom can be in our analysis. The repeating modality <
er indicates ACON. The General Symptoms in this case, thirsty and < warm
d by many remedies in the homeopathic materia medica. However only
has been recorded because we are only interested in those remedies which
symptoms of the Chief Complaint - ACON., BELL., and PULS., and out of
. matches.

ase, for burning pain in throat there are a number of other remedies which
in throat, but we have *only* recorded those remedies (ACON. and BELL.)
the stronger Local Symptom of throbbing pain in ears - because the ear
case are much more pronounced at three underlines. The throat symptom is

mportant point regarding matching remedies to the symptoms. When we
g symptoms in the case with a group of remedies clearly corresponding to
to analyze less important symptoms it is safe to record only those remedies
trongest symptoms.

ere is no great differentiation between the strength of the symptoms, more
lved in matching all the remedies to each of the main symptoms in the case,
remedy becomes clear. Based upon these guiding perspectives of case
the following written assignment.

Errata

Page 56:

Line 4:   (3) Throbbing pains in chest   *should read:* (3) Throbbing pains in ears

Line 40:   Burning pains in throat   *should be moved 12 spaces to the left margin*

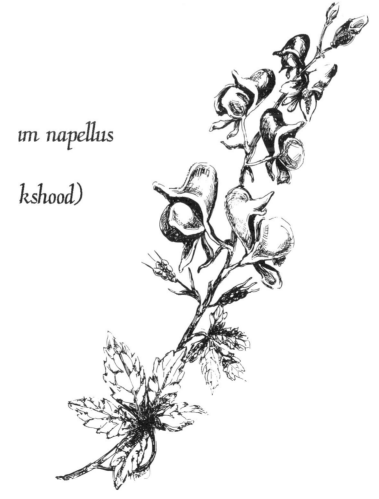

m napellus

kshood)

WRITTEN ASSIGNMENT

Read the following case data and give the name of the remedy which best matches all of the symptoms. Refer to both the cold remedies on pp. 105 - 107 TEXT and the appropriate TEXT chart for the answer. Use the method of writing the abbreviations of the remedies next to the symptoms they match, to simplify your task. You may wish to refer to the TEXT materia medica to confirm your decision and learn more about the remedy.

1. CHIEF COMPLAINT - A Cold with Burning Sore Throat
    LOCAL SYMPTOMS
    (2) Burning Sore Throat
    (3) > hot drinks
    (1) Watery mucus discharge from nose
    (2) < after midnight
    (1) Mucus irritates nose
    (1) Sneezing
    GENERAL SYMPTOMS
    (3) Chilly
    (3) Thirsty for sips of warm drinks.

What is the remedy?

2. CHIEF COMPLAINT - A Cold with Dizziness
    ETIOLOGY - patient moved to a warm climate in the middle of a cold winter.
    ONSET - developed slowly.
    LOCAL SYMPTOMS
    (3) Dizziness
    (2) Headache
    (1) Watery discharge from nose

    GENERAL SYMPTOMS
    (3) Feels tired and heavy
    (2) Thirstless
    (1) Chills up and down spine

What is the remedy?
Read this remedy in the Materia Medica if you have not already done so.

3. CHIEF COMPLAINT - A Cold
    LOCAL SYMPTOMS
    (3) Thick yellow mucus easily expectorated
    (2) > cool open air
    (1) Low grade fever
    (1) > cold applications

GENERAL SYMPTOMS
> (2) > cool open air, cool temperatures
> Thirstless

MENTAL/EMOTIONAL SYMPTOMS
> (3) Weeping often
> (3) Desires company - does not want to be
>   alone.
>   (Normally she is fine when left alone)

What is the remedy?

Analysis of Multiple Symptom Cases

In covering the flu, colds, sore throats, coughs and earaches, we notice in the TEXT and Syllabus that each type of illness has a section or differential portrayed by itself. This is helpful in illustrating how remedies relate to each specific illness. We come across two types of cases in homeopathic analysis of acute complaints.

> A. The type of case where the Chief Complaint has one outstanding
> symptom of focus.
> Example [1]
> CHIEF COMPLAINT - Earache
> LOCAL SYMPTOM
> > (2) Sticking pains in ear
> > > (1) < heat
>
> GENERAL SYMPTOM
> > (1) < heat

This is a simplified, relatively easy case. Your initial attempts in case analysis will usually be easier and more understandable if the case is of this type.

> B. The type of case in which the Chief Complaint has numerous interrelated
> symptoms.
> Example [2]
> CHIEF COMPLAINT - A Cold
> ONSET - sudden
> LOCAL SYMPTOMS
> > (3) Earache - throbbing pain in ear
> > > (1) < noise
> > (2) Burning pain in throat
> > > (2) < right side
> > (2) Nose congested - bloody mucus
> > Dry cough
> > > > sitting up
>
> GENERAL SYMPTOMS
> > (3) Flushed face
> > (2) Thirstless
> > (1) Restless

---

1 The symptoms of this case match Chamomilla / Cham.
2 The symptoms of this case strongly correspond to Belladonna / Bell.

In the above example the Cold is comprised of an earache, sore throat, congested nose and a cough. In treating the flu, colds, sore throats, coughs and earaches, we notice in the TEXT and Syllabus that each type of illness has a section or differential portrayed by itself. This illustrates how remedies relate to each specific illness. It must be remembered, however, that homeopathy looks at the totality of symptoms. It is holistic in the truest sense of the word. Obviously, as in the above example, the Cold with earache, sore throat, stuffed nose and cough are part of one person's symptom picture (a Cold) and these symptoms of the Cold are interrelated.

Multiple Symptom Cases - Organizing the Data

Note how the case data has been organized in the previous case.[1] Due care has been given towards listing the symptoms in descending order of intensity. In situations where two symptoms exist which have an equal number of underlines, a decision needs to be made which symptom ought to be considered first. The symptom listed first will tend to be given greater emphasis in case analysis. Ultimately this decision will be based upon the following considerations, together with your own personal sense of which symptom is more important.

If one of the symptoms has a stronger modality underneath it, list that one first.
    Example:
    In the above case   (2) Burning pain in throat
                         (2)< right side
                         (2) Nose congested - bloody mucus
                            > sitting up
The sore throat and congested nose have equal intensity of underlines yet we place the sore throat first because its modality has two underlines, whereas the modality of the congested nose has none.

If one of the symptoms matches the description in your homeopathic reference books more clearly, list that one first.

If one of the symptoms strikes you as being strange or uniquely peculiar list that one first.
            Example of a uniquely peculiar symptom:
                (2) Sore throat
                (2) < drinking liquids

A sore throat worse from drinking liquids is uniquely peculiar. One would assume usually that a sore throat would be relieved from liquids. Moreover there are only a few homeopathic remedies in the entire materia medica which match this symptom. Try to be attentive in casetaking and analysis so as to recognize these rare and unique symptoms. By emphasizing them in case analysis it will often help narrow down your search to a few remedies.

Multiple Symptom Cases - Analysis Guidelines

The way to success in case analysis lies in developing a sense of which are the important symptoms in a case, out of a mass of data. Each case is unique. You've got to be flexible. Try to adapt yourself to each particular situation. In some cases there may be no outstanding Mental/Emotional Symptoms. Many cases will have no valuable Etiology or Onset. In other

---

1 Also review back to Format for Recording Symptoms p. 39 Syllabus.

cases the General Symptoms may be vague, while the Local and Mental/Emotional Symptoms are clear. Always go to analyze the strongest symptoms in each case, which should be apparent when the case data has been properly perceived and organized.

WRITTEN ASSIGNMENT

4. Find the remedy for the following case. Rewrite or copy the symptoms listed and record your analysis by placing the abbreviations of the remedies to the right of the matching symptoms. Try to get the whole case on one side of a page and record the symptoms closer to the left hand margin to allow ample space for writing the remedy abbreviations.
In your answer include the full and abbreviated name of the correct remedy, suggest a potency, and write down the directions for frequency of usage.

Case Story: Influenza - 10-year-old boy

A boy 10 years old went on a camping trip to Canada where the weather was much cooler and damper. Toward the last week of the trip he developed a cold, which got increasingly worse and went into the chest. Unfortunately he was not given a homeopathic remedy in the early stages. Dulcamara or Anas Barbariae Hepatis et Cordis may have reduced the chances of the flu developing. But now he returns home with symptoms of the flu.

CHIEF COMPLAINT - Influenza

LOCAL SYMPTOMS
        Influenza with aching pains
            (3) Aching pains
                (2) > movement
                (1) > hot baths
            (2) Sore Throat with hoarse voice
                (2) > warm tea
            (2) Expectoration of thick yellow mucus
            (1) Dry Cough
            (1) Slight fever

GENERAL SYMPTOMS
            (3) Restless
            (2) Chilly

LESSON 6

Locating Hard to Find Symptoms

What do we do during a case analysis when we cannot find an important symptom in the specific TEXT chapter, chart or the materia medica?

Another place to look for the symptom is in the TEXT Mini-Repertory pp. 249 - 255. This mini-repertory is a simplified listing of symptoms and the remedies that match them. It has been compiled especially for use with the acute conditions covered in the TEXT. The mini-repertory only lists the remedies in the TEXT and is not complete. For example it does not list Rhus tox. Be that as it may, it still is a valuable tool.

How to use the Mini-Repertory:
1. Locate the symptom in the Mini-Repertory.

2. Examine the remedies listed for that symptom and write them in on your case analysis next to the symptom.

3. The remedies listed in CAPITAL letters indicate they figure more prominently for that symptom. Therefore they are given more consideration. However, one still considers the remedies not in capitals.

NOTE: Turn to p. 252 in the Mini-Repertory to the section # 5. Complaints, A. Location. While, on occasion, this section might help guide you in case analysis - generally the use of this section is not advisable.

If an important symptom is not to be found in the TEXT anywhere, then it may be necessary to look for it in BOERICKE'S Repertory pp. 689 - 979. Always try to find it in the TEXT first. BOERICKE'S Repertory contains infinitely more material but is much more complex.

Finding a Symptom in Boericke

There are two ways to find a symptom in BOERICKE:

The first way is to turn to the Repertory Index, pp. 983 - 992. The index is an excellent way to locate a symptom by the name of its complaint. One endeavors to locate the name of the complaint in this index. However many of the complaints listed in this index are listed by their diagnosis, using medical terminology which may require a medical dictionary in order to be understood.

Example: Someone has a sore throat with loss of voice. Loss of voice is listed on p. 983 of the index as Aphonia. By referring to the page number for the complaint, one finds the symptoms listed there with the remedies.

The other way is to search through the actual chapters and subheadings of the repertory itself. The chapters in order of their appearance are: Mind, Head, Eyes, Ears, Nose, Face, Mouth, Tongue, Taste, Gums, Teeth, Throat, Stomach, Abdomen, Urinary System, Male Sexual System, Female Sexual System, Circulatory System, Locomotor System, Respiratory System, Skin, Fever, Nervous System, Generalities, and Modalities.

Once the symptom sought is found, there will be a list of remedies. A number of the remedies listed will not be in most remedy kits. The remedies in italics will be the ones more strongly indicated for that symptom. It is good to gain familiarity with BOERICKE. At the same time it is practical wisdom to first become well grounded and familiar with the use of the basic remedies which are in most home remedy kits. Expanding too rapidly to the full range of all the homeopathic remedies with premature attempts at advanced case analysis could be at cross purposes with one's learning.

WRITTEN ASSIGNMENT

1. Find the remedies listed for the following symptoms in the TEXT mini-repertory, and list them by their abbreviation. Underline those remedies which appear in capitals.

> A. Desires cold food
> B. Anxious expression

2. Find the remedies listed for the following symptoms in BOERICKE. However, list only those remedies which are italicized. List the remedies by their abbreviation and underline those remedies which appear in italics. Use the Repertory Index for locating the complaint.[1]

> A. Lumbago (Loins)
> B. Constipation (from gastric derangements)

Coughs

Coughs can be tricky to analyze. Some coughs have an obvious trait. Distinguishing a dry cough (Bryonia), from a cough with loose rattling mucus (Hepar sulph), is not difficult. Some coughs will definitely be made worse or better from particular temperatures.

However let's take an example of a not so obvious cough case. Suppose we are working to find a remedy to matching a cough that is the Chief Complaint in a case. Suppose the cough is dry but does not have any other outstanding features. In this situation we examine the General Symptoms to see how the physical appearance, reaction to temperature, and thirst, etc., figure with the cough symptoms.

What if the remedy is still unclear? Then we examine the other symptoms in the case which are strongly underlined. After coming up with several remedies or a remedy which matches the other symptoms, one can then refer back to see how these remedies match the cough. In some cases it is necessary to read in more detail about the remedies in BOERICKE to make a final decision. A hint for simplifying our referral to BOERICKE is to find the specific heading for the symptom. For instance a cough is listed under the Respiratory heading under Bryonia in BOERICKE. Look at Bryonia in BOERICKE now and see where the cough information is given.

---

[1] If you happen to encounter the remedy abbreviation, 'Sul' in BOERICKE, it means SULPH or SULPHUR. This is one of the minor incongruities which occasionally appear in the books.

WRITTEN ASSIGNMENT

3. If you are having a hard time finding a remedy to match a cough which is the Chief Complaint, what steps may be taken to find the remedy?

READING ASSIGNMENT

Read Coughs in the TEXT pp. 110 - 112. As you read each cough remedy, find it and study it in the Chart on pp. 114 - 127.

WRITTEN ASSIGNMENT

4. The Aconite cough is worse from entering a warm room. How does this differ from the Rumex cough?

5. Describe the Spongia cough, utilizing the more complete description from the TEXT materia medica.

6. Describe the Kali Bichromicum cough giving a detailed account of the expectoration from BOERICKE p. 364.

7. Analyze the following case story. Rewrite the symptom data listing it in the proper format. Place the abbreviation of matching remedies next to each symptom. Give the name of the correct remedy and suggestions for the potency and frequency of usage. You may find it useful to refer back to Recommended Frequency of Usage on p. 16 of this Syllabus.

Note: The Chief Complaint in this case is - A Cold.

CASE STORY: Cold - a girl nine years old.
My friend's daughter has quite a cold. Here are the symptoms elicited:
Her nose is stuffed with thick yellow mucus (3) which seems to be worse at night (2). Her nose unclogs and runs during the day when she sits out on the porch (3). She has been coughing up some yellow mucus (2). Her cough seems improved when sitting on the porch. She is upset that she may miss her friend's birthday party and has been crying about that (2). On examining her tongue, I notice it is coated white (2) and her lips are dry (1). She is not especially thirsty.

Earaches

READING ASSIGNMENT

Read pp. 112 - 113 in TEXT. As you read each earache remedy, find it and study it in the chart pp. 114 - 127. Read the supplementary material in the Syllabus which follows.

Earaches, which are commonly indicators of ear infections, are most often seen in children. The most common type of ear infection is known as Otitis Media, which means that there is an infection of the middle ear, on the inside of the ear drum. If untreated, the infection inside the ear could build up and eventually rupture the ear drum, causing a discharge of pus. If the ear drum ruptures, normally the ear drum heals rapidly after that. However, the infection could travel towards the brain with very serious consequences, but this is an extremely rare occurrence.

Conventional medicine treats these acute ear infections with antibiotics and, if they keep recurring often, ventilating tubes are put in the ear drums. However, antibiotics, as research and experience are showing, do not always resolve ear infections. There are studies which show that their effect is doubtful. Additionally, antibiotics weaken the immune system, the natural defenses of a person's health. Therefore the child with a mild ear infection who is treated with antibiotics becomes more prone to recurring infections because the immune system is further weakened. The use of tubes in the ear drum does allow fluids in the inner ear to drain out and temporarily improves hearing. However, the tubes can cause scar tissue on the ear drum and are not a long term solution to the problem.

Anyone having chronically recurring ear infections should seek professional help under the care of a homeopathic physician. Homeopathy is a reliable and effective means for resolving these infections. You will usually be able to resolve earaches with the remedies found in most home remedy kits. But always seek professional help where there has been a history of recurring earaches or infections. In some cases the underlying causes of these infections are from the side effects of vaccinations. An experienced homeopath is needed to remove this underlying disturbance in the vital force.

When analyzing an earache case, it is suggested that you first examine the TEXT differential for earaches. Then go to the following Syllabus differential where more complete information or confirmation is needed.

Frequency of Usage for Earaches

Earache pain can be intense and discomforting. If your carefully selected remedy does not show signs of relieving intense pain within 30 minutes, the remedy could be incorrect. Another possibility is that the remedy could be the right choice but its potency is incorrect, usually it is too low for the intensity of the earache.[1]

---

[1]In cases of intense pain, when the remedy is correct but the potency is too low, one usually notices a short-lived improvement. This is a possible sign that the remedy has been given in too low a potency.

In cases of intense pain, the correct remedy will usually show signs of relief within the first 30 minutes. It is not necessary to wait 12 hours before changing the remedy or potency in this situation. In this case one is justified to change the remedy or potency within 30 minutes if there are no signs of relief.

When selecting another remedy, always make your choice carefully. Make an effort to study the symptoms carefully and read the appropriate differential and materia medica. By making the effort to study the case and the appropriate materia medica, you will be deepening your working knowledge of homeopathy. The remedy you select will also have a better chance of being correct.

Sometimes the intensity of an earache will warrant a higher potency remedy, i.e.. 12C, 30X or 30C. In such an instance the correct remedy may have been given in too low a potency, i.e.. 3X or 6X, to have much effect. In this situation how does one know whether it is the potency which is too low, or whether it is the wrong remedy choice?

If when restudying the symptoms another remedy seems to figure as a good possibility, that could be a sign that a change of remedy is needed. If the symptoms strongly match the original remedy with no other remedy appearing close, and if the original remedy was given in low potency, i.e.. 3X or 6X, that is a sign that the earache may require a higher potency of the same remedy, i.e.. 30C, especially if there was some improvement after giving the remedy the first time.

Example: 11-month Teething Infant with Earache
      CHIEF COMPLAINT - Earache

      LOCAL SYMPTOMS
            (3) Infant screaming in great pain
                (2) < warm room
                (1) < 10 p.m. - 11 p.m.
            (2) Pulling at ears
            (2) Teething

      GENERAL SYMPTOMS
            (3) One side of face is red other side is pale

      M/E
            (3) Great irritability
            (3) Child is thrashing in bed

This case clearly corresponds to the remedy Chamomilla. (See Chamomilla in the Earache Differential on p. 67 to affirm that the symptoms match strongly). Chamomilla 3X is given once. The report after 30 minutes is that there were a few minutes of improvement after taking the remedy, which did not last. The symptoms are now the same as before. Upon reviewing the symptoms it is concluded that Chamomilla is still the best choice. In this situation a higher potency of the same remedy is given - Chamomilla 30C.[1] The symptoms then subside and the infant falls asleep peacefully. 30C is a high enough potency to yield some results if the remedy choice is correct. If the symptoms persist and your well selected remedy(ies) do not resolve the earache, see a homeopathic physician.

---

1 If a higher potency (i.e. 30C) of the same remedy is not readily available, the technique of 'plussing' outlined on p. 53 Syllabus may be employed.

Caution: avoid taking or giving high potency homeopathic remedies on your own, i.e.. 200C, IM, 10M etc. These high potencies should only be given by an experienced homeopath.

Having given the correct homeopathic remedy for an earache, the first symptoms to go are the pain and somewhat later, fever. The inflammation and fluid commonly take a few days to subside. If the pain and fever persist, see a homeopathic physician.

Earache Differential

Chamomilla / Cham.
Violent pains worse warmth and warm stuffy rooms. Onset is fast or slow. Worse 9 p.m. - 12 a.m. Children pulling on ear, screaming, crying, fussy, thrashing, fretful, irritable, angry, in great pain. One side of the face may be red, while the other side is pale. Capriciousness, child does not know what it wants. Will not let you examine ear.

Pulsatilla / Puls.
Develops a few days after a cold, with thick yellow-greenish discharge from ear. Severe throbbing pain. Wishes to be held and comforted. Whiny, better being carried. Ear feels stopped up. Pain typically worse at night and in a warm room. Kicks off covers in sleep. Better open air. One side of the face may be red while the other side is pale.

Belladonna / Bell.
Pains come and go suddenly with intensity. Onset is sudden. Especially right ear is affected, though not exclusively so. Worse at 9 p.m. at night. Better warmth. Throbbing pains. Pupils dilated. Fever with red flushed face. Face is red and warm to touch and may be inflamed. Aggravated by touch, light and noise. Dryness of mouth with aversion to water or thirst for cold water.

Indented tongue. Notice the tongue's edge which bears the 'indented' imprint of where the tongue rests against the teeth. The extent of the imprints can vary considerably. With complaints requiring Mercurius, one often sees an indented tongue. Pulsatilla also can have this type of tongue but not as prominently. Other common remedies which can have an indented tongue are Arsenicum alb, and Rhus tox.

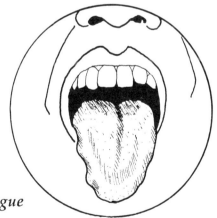

Indented Tongue

Mercurius viv. or sol. / Merc.
Sharp stabbing pain in ear - can be a severe earache. Discharge of pus coming out of ear. Roaring in ears. Worse heat, worse cold, typically worse warmth and warmth of bed. Worse at night. Swollen lymph glands. Offensive breath and puffiness of tongue which can be indented. (see illustration). Can have an oily or offensive perspiration on the head.

Hepar sulph / Hep.

Chilly sensitive to drafts. Irritable though not as much as Chamomilla. Sharp pains in ear. Whole side of face sensitive to touch. Sensitivity to winds, drafts. Better warmth. For middle and late stages of ear infections espccially with impending pus discharge. Thick creamy and offensive discharge. Worse at night. Mastoiditis - inflammation of the bone behind the ear, a potentially serious condition for which you should see a homeopathic physician.

Silicea / Sil.

Recurring earaches in weak frail child. Promotes healing of ear drum. For middle to late stages of ear infections. A picture of mildness, whimpering, physical weakness and tiredness. Chilly seeks warm covering. Itching sensations in ear.

Kali muriaticum / Kali mur.

Specific for deafness or slowly progressing deafness following otitis media - will often yield to this remedy. This remedy clears the eustachian tube. Specific for earache flying in an airplane caused by change of air pressure and blocked eustachian tube.
Kali muriaticum, known as Kali mur. is a homeopathic tissue salt. Homeopathic tissue salts are available at most health food stores.

Causticum / Caust.

Roaring, buzzing, re-echoing sounds. Earache with catarrh of eustachian tube. Etiology - wind blowing in ears.

BEYOND FIRST AID - (Supplement to the TEXT advice.)
See a homeopathic physician in cases of severe earache, where the bony area behind the ear is tender (a sign of mastoiditis), and in any cases where the earache or discharge lasts longer than one week.

WRITTEN ASSIGNMENT

8. Name the remedy which is specific for earaches while flying in an airplane.
What does this remedy do to relieve the pain?
What use may this remedy have for a person recovering from the effects of ear infections?

9. What is a children's remedy for ear infections, where there is great pain which is worse from warmth? The child is classically irritable, fretful, and is thrashing about. Describe one dental use of this remedy. (May be found in the TEXT).

10. Name an ear infection remedy that has fever with intense onset and pains. The pains are throbbing and the whole side of the face may be red and warm. In spite of this the pain is better from warmth. There is great sensitivity to touch, light, and noise.

---

* * * STOP * * *

Before you continue with the next lesson, send to your instructor your responses to all of the written assignments from Lessons 5 and 6. Is everything clear to you about the material covered thus far? If you have any questions now is the time to send them to your instructor.

Notes:

LESSON 7

Case Analysis Hints

In case analysis these hints will be used continually so bear them in mind.

1. When matching symptoms to the remedy, never or rarely will *all* of the symptoms of that remedy be present in a case. The guiding rule is to base the decision on what symptoms *match* the remedy as opposed to what symptoms are not present. In other words approach it in a *positive* way.

Example: A Hepar sulph earache case in which the person is worse from drafts, complains of stitching pains and is sensitive to touch. However, the person is not displaying pronounced irritability. Hepar sulph is known for irritability. It is correct to give Hepar sulph in this case, even if some sympton(s) of Hepar sulph are absent.

As we see, when matching symptoms to the remedy, it is unusual to find every symptom matching. However any strong modalities or General Symptoms in the case should not contradict the general indications of the remedy.

Therefore consider if the above example of earache was not sensitive to drafts and was definitely worse from heat. In examining the remedy Hepar sulph we will find it to be improved by heat. Here, a definite modality in the case does not match and in fact contradicts Hepar sulph. In this case Hepar sulph would not be considered further. The remedy would have to be an earache remedy, which is worse from heat and matches the Local Symptoms in the case as much as possible.

2. You need to have a flexible and clever mind. Not always will someone's exact words match the remedy description as it appears in the materia medica. The homeopath must accurately interpret his or her observations and what the person says in order to match closest to the remedy description.

Example: The mother says the child is cranky - there is no such word in the repertory. So you need to visualize the child's state and match it to the closest remedy description.

WRITTEN ASSIGNMENT

1. In case analysis and remedy selection describe the positive way of matching symptoms to the remedy.

Why does the homeopath need to sometimes interpret what a person says?

2. Now we have a case which, as in reality, can seem a little ambiguous. This case involves your making an effort to put the case analysis hints, mentioned above, into practice.

*Solve the following case of earache with sore throat. Find the **one curative remedy** for this case. List the symptoms clearly according to the advised format. Refer to the Sore Throat Differential in this Syllabus - Lesson 4, pp. 46-47 and in the Earache Differential in Lesson 6, pp. 67-68. Also, refer to the appropriate TEXT chapters and chart to match the symptoms. If you cannot find a symptom in the Syllabus or TEXT remedy descriptions, then look for it in the TEXT mini-repertory or BOERICKE. It may be helpful to refer to your chosen remedy in BOERICKE'S materia medica to confirm your analysis.*

Note: In actual experience, sometimes the suffering subject can report the symptoms with incorrect emphasis. This case illustrates the point. Remember the Chief Complaint in this case is the earache, and the narration which follows is not necessarily in the order in which the symptoms should be organized.

Case Story: College student with Earache and Sore Throat

CHIEF COMPLAINT - Earache

He reports that the sore throat started on the right side (1), about a week before the earache started. Now both sides of the throat are sore (1), with a burning pain (1). He is losing his voice (2). The discomfort is worse at night (3). The glands of his neck are swollen (3).
The ear pains are sometimes sharp (2) and sticking (2) and are felt in the ear on swallowing (1). The pain is worse at night (3).
He is worse from cold weather (3) and from heat (3). He is thirsty for cold drinks and is irritable (1).

READING ASSIGNMENT

Hepar sulph Materia Medica.
Read Hepar sulph in the TEXT materia medica on p. 263 and, if available, in your remedy kit brochure.
Read Hepar sulph in BOERICKE on pp. 325 - 327, scanning the material by placing emphasis on finding the same symptoms that are in the TEXT. Read the modalities carefully.
Note: Suppuration means the formation and discharge of pus.

WRITTEN ASSIGNMENT

Hepar sulph Materia Medica
3. Is the Hepar sulph case warm blooded or chilly?

4. What environmental conditions relating to weather and temperature can bring on a Hepar sulph complaint, or aggravate it?

5. What temperature improves Hepar sulph?

6. In any Hepar sulph illness, regardless of whether it is a sore throat, boils, or earache,etc., describe the sensitivity of the Hepar sulph person.

7. What is the mood that typifies the Hepar sulph state?

8. In the case of a skin boil, which remedy taken in low potencies, such as 3X, 6X, 3C, 4C, 5C, will encourage the formation and discharge of pus to resolve the boil?

9. Write the abbreviation for Hepar sulph.

The remedies in most home remedy kits are Polychrests - medicines with many uses. Let us turn together to Arsenicum in BOERICKE pp. 79 - 83. As can be noticed, Arsenicum is a remedy for colds, influenzas, sore throats, coughs, earaches, headaches, fever and many other symptoms. In our TEXT Dr. Panos has simplified our initial homeopathic study. We cannot find her listing Arsenicum for cough or earaches; yet if we look in BOERICKE we will see Arsenicum also having coughs and earaches, though not prominently.

Homeopathy for Stomach and Bowel Problems

In Chapter 7 of the TEXT, Remedies for Stomach and Bowel Problems - there are remedy differentials for Indigestion, Nausea and Vomiting, Diarrhea, Gas, Constipation and Hemorrhoids. It is not uncommon for several of these complaints to be present in a single person. For example, a man can have indigestion with nausea, vomiting and diarrhea. In this case, as we have learned in Lesson 5, we naturally consider the strongest symptoms first. By glancing through the remedy differential for each of these complaints it is not surprising to see some of the same remedies again and again.

As we cover these complaints, supplementary material is provided in the Syllabus. In the study of homeopathy one finds that no one book contains all of the information. The positive perspective toward this is that by reading about the same remedy from different sources, we learn and remember it more completely.

READING ASSIGNMENT

Study pp. 128 - 129, Indigestion, in the TEXT. As you read each indigestion remedy, find it and study it on the chart on pp. 139 - 149. Read the Indigestion Differential that follows in the Syllabus as a supplement to the TEXT.

Indigestion Differential

Cinchona officinalis / China / Chin.
Painful distension temporarily relieved by belching. The belches can have a sour or bitter taste. Flatulence smells offensive. Slow digestion and a tendency to fainting. The food does not digest, it lies a long time in the stomach causing belching and could be vomited undigested.

Carbo vegetabilis / Carbo veg. / Carb-v.

The belching can have a rancid taste with burning pains in the stomach. There can be cramping pains which cause the person to bend double.

Ignatia / Ign.

Be on the look out for sighing in the patient. The patient will not tell you he or she sighs. It is an elusive kind of breathing which has to be observed.

Nux vomica / Nux-v.

Related to the etiology of mental overwork or an overworking business executive type of lifestyle. Overindulgence in coffee, alcohol, tobacco or drugs. Psychologically the person is irritable. The gastric disturbances characteristically do not begin right after eating, but come on 30 minutes to several hours after eating. Base of the tongue may have yellowish discoloration. Chilly and worse from exposure to cold weather.

Pulsatilla / Puls.

Tongue is coated with a thick white fur. A bad taste in the mouth as if from the food in the stomach. Acidity and heartburn. Belchings tasting of food. Dyspepsia from fatty food, pork and pastry. The person may be tearful. Worse in the evening.

Sulphur / Sulph.

Indigestion with a bitter or sour taste in the mouth. Putrid belches. Sour vomiting. Hungry at night but a small amount of food fills up the patient. Worse from starchy foods. Milk increases acidity. Desires sweets, which cause a sour stomach and heartburn. Burning pains. Aversion to bathing.

WRITTEN ASSIGNMENT

10. Describe the Carbo veg. indigestion.

11. Which remedy has gastric disturbances which begin several hours after eating?
Describe the body temperature of this remedy.

12. Which remedy has indigestion which is made worse from milk, sweets, and starchy foods?
Describe the sensation this remedy is known to have in the feet at night in bed. Refer to the TEXT materia medica.

13. Which indigestion remedy is known for having a bad taste in the mouth?
Describe the mood of this remedy.
Describe the thirst of this remedy.

READING ASSIGNMENT

Study Nausea, Vomiting and Gas, p. 130 to the bottom of p. 132 in the TEXT. Find the remedies discussed in the chart on pp. 139 - 149, and read.

Consider Cocculus as an addition to the Nausea and Vomiting remedies.

Cocculus indicus / Cocculus
The nausea and vomiting of this remedy are easy to recognize. It is specific for travel sickness whether in a car, airplane or boat. The symptoms are often accompanied by dizziness. Cocculus also is specific for the effects of jet lag and nerve weakness from loss of sleep.

An added differentiation between the gas of Carbo veg. and Lycopodium:
Carbo veg. gas tends to be more in the stomach. It is felt more from the navel up and is associated with belching. Lycopodium gas occurs more in the intestines and is felt more below the navel. There is more passing of flatus.

WRITTEN ASSIGNMENT

14. What remedy would come to mind for a vomiting person who has a clean tongue?
Describe the intestinal pains of this remedy.
Describe the saliva of this remedy.

15. What remedy would come to mind in this situation? A child is nauseous and is vomiting. The mother is not sure what the cause may have been. Upon your inquiring about the thirst of the child the mother sadly reports the child has been desiring cold water, but after a little while vomits it.

16. What remedy would come to mind in this situation? An elderly man is vomiting. His energy is totally wiped out and he is chilly. He feels better from warmth and is covered with clammy perspiration.

17. Which nausea remedy comes to mind for these symptoms? A businessman is observed in front of a fast food restaurant. He has intense abdominal cramps and is doubled over, pressing his abdomen.
What temperature would tend to relieve this condition?

18. Upon buying ripe papayas, which were on sale, Allen ravenously ate one, only to find halfway through that he swallowed a portion which was spoiled. What remedy resolved Allen's subsequent nausea, vomiting, and diarrhea?
Describe the stomach pains and thirst which are characteristic of this remedy.

19. Which remedy can have an upset stomach, nausea and an unfulfilled desire to vomit? From the TEXT materia medica write out the modalities of this remedy.

20. What remedy has vomiting right after eating too much food? Describe the characteristic appearance of the tongue in this remedy. Find the description in BOERICKE.

21. Which remedy has gas and belching 1/2 hour after eating?
What is the common name for this remedy?

READING ASSIGNMENT

Carbo vegetabilis Materia Medica
Read Carbo vegetabilis in the TEXT materia medica on p. 261 and, if available, in your remedy kit brochure.
Read Carbo vegetabilis in BOERICKE on pp. 169 - 172, scanning the material by placing emphasis on finding the same symptoms in the TEXT. Read the modalities carefully.

WRITTEN ASSIGNMENT

Carbo vegetabilis Materia Medica
23. Describe the body temperature of a Carbo veg. case.

24. What kinds of foods would especially aggravate a Carbo veg. case?

25. After a Carbo veg. person eats, describe the symptoms that develop in the stomach and intestines.

26. If a Carbo veg. case has stomach gas, how would belching affect the condition?

READING ASSIGNMENT

Phosphorus Materia Medica.
Read Phosphorus in the TEXT materia medica on p. 267 and, if available, in your remedy kit brochure.
Read Phosphorus in BOERICKE on pgs. 507-511, scanning the material by placing emphasis on finding the same symptoms in the TEXT. Read the modalities carefully.

WRITTEN ASSIGNMENT

Phosphorus Materia Medica.
27. In a case of Phosphorus nausea and vomiting, when are the ice cold drinks vomited?

28. What pain typifies Phosphorus?

29. What temperature generally improves Phosphorus?

30. Phosphorus suits states of weakened blood vessels and hemorrhages. Give 3 types of bleeding which Phosphorus could help.

31. Write the abbreviation for Phosphorus.

READING ASSIGNMENT

Study Constipation in the TEXT pp. 132 - 135. As you read each constipation remedy, find it and study it in the chart on pp. 139 - 149. Then study the supplementary material that follows in the Syllabus.

Constipation Differential

Nux vomica / Nux-v.

A widely indicated remedy for constipation characterized by a continual desire and urge to have a bowel movement with the bowel movement being incomplete. If the person has no desire to go, then Nux vomica is probably not the remedy. Constipation worse in the mornings and after dinner.

Phosphorus / Phos.

Constipation with long hard slender stools, that look like a dog's. There is much straining during a bowel movement.

Veratrum album / Verat.

The constipation of this remedy is characterized by a build up of stool at the rectum. The upper part of the intestines are not constipated. The constipation is an inactivity in the lower part of the intestines. The stool is large, hard and dark. Could break out in a sweat while straining. Weakness after stool.

WRITTEN ASSIGNMENT

32. What constipation remedy comes to mind for getting a person off dependence on laxatives?
Describe the constipation characteristic of this remedy. What is the optimal time for taking this remedy?

33. A young man is constipated. He is tall, slender and had has red hair. He is having a hard time describing his constipation. Finally upon being questioned as to the appearance of his stool he says it is long, hard and thin like a dog's.
What is the remedy?
List a main characteristic of the vomiting of this remedy.

READING ASSIGNMENT

Study Diarrhea in the TEXT pp. 135 - 136. As you read each diarrhea remedy, find it and study it in the chart on pp. 139 - 149. Then read the supplementary material in the syllabus which follows.

Diarrhea Differential

Arsenicum album / Ars.
Diarrhea expelled in small quantities with offensive odor, followed by great weakness. There is often restlessness and can have burning pain in the rectum. Great thirst for small quantities often. Intolerance of pain.

Veratrum album / Verat.
Similar to Arsenicum but has larger quantities of diarrhea. Profuse and watery diarrhea. No restlessness. Great thirst for large quantities of cold water. Pain in abdomen before stool. Cold sweat.

Aloe
Lumpy watery stools. Griping pains in the lower abdomen and around the navel before and during stool. The pains are better after stool. After stool there is weakness and perspiration. With Aloe there is a feeling of uncertainty that diarrhea will escape if gas comes out of the rectum.

Sulphur / Sulph.
Diarrhea with rectal soreness and itching.

Painless Diarrheas

Cinchona officinalis / China / Chin.
Painless diarrhea that smells like a corpse. Worse at night after eating, with exhaustion and debility. Thirsty for small quantities often like Arsenicum, but painless, no burning. Summer diarrhea.

Phosphorus / Phos.
Chronic painless diarrhea. Involuntary escape of diarrhea with flatus as with Aloes. Stools often contain undigested food. Weak, gone sensation in stomach.

WRITTEN ASSIGNMENT

Answer the following questions. Refer first to the TEXT chapter and chart, then to the Syllabus.

34. What is the remedy for this diarrhea case?
Profuse, watery stools (2), with weakness following stools (1). Pains in the abdomen before (2) and during stool (2) and better after stool (3). Diarrhea is uncontrollably passed when flatulence is emitted (3).
Find this remedy in BOERICKE and note the symptoms italicized in the Rectum paragraph.

35. Name the remedy which best suits this case:
Profuse gushing watery stools (3). The stool smells bad (3). A feeling of weakness in the abdomen after stool (2). The patient has intestinal gas which makes sounds in the abdomen (2). There are colicky cramps in the abdomen (2).

36. Name the painless diarrhea remedy characterized by exhaustion and weakness. The stool has a cadaverous odor. Describe the thirst of this remedy.

37. Describe the difference between the Arsenicum and Veratrum album Diarrheas.

READING ASSIGNMENT

Cinchona officinalis / China Materia Medica.
Read China in your remedy kit brochure if you have one and in BOERICKE pp. 207 - 210, by scanning the material placing emphasis on the stomach symptoms and the modalities.

WRITTEN ASSIGNMENT

China Materia Medica.
38. Loss of blood, diarrhea, and a bout of influenza are potential causes to make the China feel _ .
(Complete the sentence).

39. What environmental conditions make a China case worse?

40. What modalities improve a China case?

41. Write the abbreviation for this remedy.

READING ASSIGNMENT

Study Hemorrhoids in the TEXT on pp. 137 - 138. As you read each hemorrhoid remedy, find it and study it in the chart on pp. 139 - 149. Then study the Hemorrhoids Differential which follows in the TEXT.

Hemorrhoids Differential

Arnica / Arn.
Suited to cases where there is a bruised sensation upon touching the hemorrhoids. Specific for hemorrhoids after childbirth.

Aesculus / Aesc.
The most common remedy for hemorrhoids, taken internally and used as an external application. Sensation of fullness in the region of the liver. Dryness and burning. May or may not bleed. Feeling of splinters or sticks in the rectum.

Hamamelis / Ham.
Bleeding hemorrhoids. The flow of blood is copious. Excessive soreness. Commonly used as an external application.

Collinsonia / Coll.

Continuous bleeding. Suited for pregnant women. Sensation of sticks in rectum. Constipation with large stools.

Sulphur / Sulph.

Hemorrhoids with constipation. Dislikes heat. Itching about anus; worse at night.

Nux vomica / Nux-v.

People who overindulge in food and drink. Constipated. Chilly. Hemorrhoids are better from cold application.

Nitric acidum / Nit-ac.

Fissures in the rectum bleeding easily, causing splinter-like pains. Pain is worse when moving bowels.

Aloe

Hemorrhoids protrude like a bunch of grapes. Bleed easily. Better cold water. Discharge of jelly from anus.

WRITTEN ASSIGNMENT

42. Solve the following gastro-intestinal case. Rewrite the symptoms with underlines in the proper format as given on p. 39 Syllabus. In your analysis place the abbreviation of the remedy to the right of the symptom it matches.

In some cases it may be necessary to translate the symptoms from one's observation or the suffering subject's own words, to suit the description in the Syllabus, TEXT or BOERICKE. Make an effort to do this in this case. Try to use all of the symptoms in the analysis. Homeopaths must be creative and wise in the interpretation of a case. Referral to the remedy being considered in the TEXT materia medica or BOERICKE may be helpful to confirm the analysis.

Case Story: Indigestion
Anne, a busy young housewife with two children and a part-time job comes complaining of indigestion (3). Her stomach has not been functioning well. She reports that there is a lot of belching after eating (2). Upon our inquiring as to whether the belching left any taste in her mouth she says it leaves a 'kind of sour taste' (1). She cannot say what is causing the condition. She does love Mexican food (2) and drinks coffee (2) to keep going. Anne also tells of her tendency toward constipation (2) and that she never seems to have a complete bowel movement. She adds that there is some feeling of nausea (2) with the indigestion. It is a warm day; however, on shaking hands we find that her hand is cold (3). We noticed she came in wearing sunglasses. During the interview it is noticed that she is hurried (2) and irritated with her 21-month-old son, who is squirming on her lap. We inquire as to the time factor when belching occurs in relation to eating. She says it is hard to tell, but it is usually not immediately after eating.

READING ASSIGNMENT

Nux vomica Materia Medica
Read Nux vomica in the TEXT materia medica on p. 267 and, if available, in your remedy kit brochure.
Read Nux vomica in BOERICKE on pp. 475 - 478, scanning the material by placing emphasis on finding the same symptoms that are in the TEXT. Read the modalities carefully.

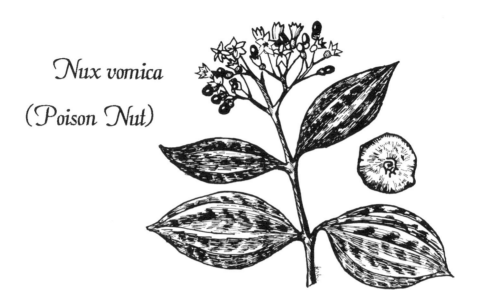

Nux vomica

(Poison Nut)

WRITTEN ASSIGNMENT

Nux vomica Materia Medica
Think of one person you know or have met who bears a resemblance to the Nux vomica type.

47. List the digestive symptoms for which Nux vomica is indicated for.

48. List the foods and substances which aggravate the Nux vomica condition.

49. Describe the temperament that typifies Nux vomica.

50. Is the Nux vomica state chilly or warm blooded?

51. What temperature aggravates a Nux vomica complaint?

LESSON 8

Homeopathy for Children

We begin our study of children's complaints with a discussion on the issue of vaccinations (immunizations). The issue of vaccinations is a controversial one. Vaccinations are administered routinely to children in the United States. Experienced homeopaths have long observed that vaccination can potentially cause a deep disturbance, altering the vital force of some people. Homeopaths term the ill effects of vaccinations, Vaccinosis. All vaccinations, but especially the DPT (Diptheria/Pertussis/Tetanus), is showing evidence of causing side effects. It is the (P) Pertussis (whooping cough) part of the DPT vaccine which is proving to be harmful. Other vaccines may not cause side effects as prominently. Also there have been questions as to the efficacy of a vaccine to create an immunity.

The topic of vaccination, if viewed superficially, appears to be homeopathic because the person is receiving a preparation from the epidemic bacteria or virus to stimulate an immunity to it. It is not really homeopathic however, because the vaccine is not selected on a basis of homeopathicity - similarity of symptoms. And it is important to recognize that the physical dose of the vaccine tends to interfere with the natural functioning of the vital force in many people.

It is a relief to know that homeopathy can usually remove the energy disturbances caused by vaccination. In children a common result of vaccination is a weakened immune system associated with chronically recurring ear infections and colds. Homeopathy can also remove the effects of vaccination in an adult after many years. The sphere of removing the effects of vaccination belongs to the homeopathic physician. The ultimate decision whether to have a child fully vaccinated, partially vaccinated, or not vaccinated at all rests in the hands of the parents. It is possible to legally refuse vaccinations for your child. See Appendix C on p. 132 of Syllabus for vital resources of information on immunizations. For those parents who wish to have their children vaccinated it is recommended that the child be under constitutional care of a homeopathic physician prior to the vaccination. If following the vaccination the child has a reaction, that reaction can be treated acutely with homeopathic remedies. Then afterwards the child continues with constitutional homeopathic treatment. By following this procedure, the harmful effects of vaccinations usually can be eliminated by homeopathy. An experienced homeopath has two approaches for removing the vaccination layer:
1. To give the vaccine potentized as a homeopathic remedy.
2. To prescribe the remedy based on the constitutional type and side effects from the vaccination.

Additionally, there are homeopathically prepared vaccines. Some studies have been made with these homeopathically prepared vaccines during epidemics and the statistics have indicated them to have a measurable degree of effectivity. However not enough scientifically conclusive studies have been made so there remain uncertainties as to the efficacy of homeopathically prepared vaccines in all cases and for how long they may remain effective. It must also be said that similar uncertainties exist for allopathic vaccinations. Also, in the homeopathic community, questions have been raised regarding the ultimate safety of routinely employing homeopathically prepared vaccines. Some homeopaths favor constitutional homeopathic treatment with acute homeopathic treatment for acute conditions that may arise, while selectively minimizing or avoiding the use of vaccines, homeopathically prepared and/or allopathic.

A research project of vast proportions is needed for vaccines. As it is not likely to happen overnight, one has to educate oneself based upon the information available and draw one's own conclusions.

Remedies for Acute Reactions Immediately Following Vaccination[1]

Ledum palustre / Ledum. / Led.
Nondescript reactions for any vaccination. However Ledum is specific for DPT vaccination. As we have learned Ledum is used for puncture wounds, wounds from sharp pointed instruments, and for poisonous insect bites.

With Ledum, the arm or leg looks bruised with ecchymosis: black and blue discoloration. The area around the vaccination may be dark, bruised, sore, achy, and infected. It does not heal well.

Hepar sulph / Hep.
When the vaccination site does not heal. Pus formation is prominent and the area is sensitive to touch.

Hypericum / Hyp.
Indicated for nondescript vaccination reactions, especially where a sharp, short pain is present. Hypericum is a remedy for injury to parts rich in nerves and puncture wounds.

Belladonna / Bell.
High fever. Whole arm or leg swells up - throbs and is hot to touch. Vaccinated area is inflamed, red and warm. Skin is flushed, hot, and dry with fever. Restless sleep - can scream out in sleep. Worse from touch, noise, light and cold air. Pupils are dilated, better from warmth.

Apis mellifica / Apis.
Vaccinated area swells up. Worse from heat - wants cold on it. May develop itchy hives - worse from heat. Face may swell up; edema of face with red rosy hue and itchy watery eyes.

Pulsatilla / Puls.
Indicated for MMR (Measles/Mumps/Rubella) vaccination. The reaction signs are these:
A morbilliform (measles-like) rash. Swelling of the glands of the neck, jaw and throat - characteristic of mumps.
Pulsatilla keynotes to look for are as follows:
Tearful - desiring company and consolation. Worse heat. Better from cold compresses, cool temperatures, being outside, moving around - can be cold sensitive.

Gelsemium / Gels.
To be thought of for acute reaction to Polio vaccination. Look for Gelsemium keynotes of muscular weakness, trembling, exhaustion, sleepiness, dizziness, and fever with chills.

Zincum metallicum / Zinc.
To be thought of for acute reaction to Polio vaccination. Restlessness at night during sleep. There is a state of irritation in the nervous system. Child wakes with a shrill irritating cry at night following vaccination. Can have restless feet.

Lathyrus sativus / Lath. (Chick pea)
To be thought of after Polio vaccination where there is paralysis particularly of the lower extremities. If in this situation - see a homeopathic physician.

---

[1] These acute reactions to vaccination remedies appear in this Lesson covering Children's Health. However, this information can be interpreted to be used for similar vaccination reactions in all age groups. Note that these remedies for acute reactions immediately following vaccination, apply more specifically to allopathic vaccinations.

The recommended potency for acute vaccination reactions is 30C. Recommended usage is 2 - 3 times a day depending on the severity of the reaction. Reduce frequency of usage with improvement. Stop taking when improvement is well established. See a homeopathic physician if condition does not improve within a few days.

NOTE: If you do not have 30C potency, a lower potency i.e., 6X, 12C or 30X, could still work if it is the correct remedy. Recommended frequency of usage for lower potencies is that they may be repeated 3 - 4 times a day which is more frequent than the 30C. Refer to the remedy vial, or your remedy kit brochure if you have one, for frequency of usage when in question.

In her coverage of complaints in babies, Dr. Panos has done a masterful job. Here she has presented the complaints in a simplified way, showing which remedy is best indicated for the symptoms *babies* exhibit. Should you be giving a homeopathic remedy to a baby, look to this chapter to find the closest matching remedy. The chart following the chapter is excellent. So be sure to use it as a reference. If, after referring to these, you are still unsure, then referring to the TEXT materia medica or to a differential earlier in the course may help. For example the earache differential earlier in the Syllabus and TEXT given in Chapter 6 provide more comprehensive information, although the chances are that you will not have to use them.

Giving Homeopathic Medicines to Infants

The recommended forms of homeopathic remedies to give to infants are: the tablets, the tiny #10 size pellets or dissolved in water. This also holds true for unconscious persons in emergency situations.

Homeopathic tablets are composed of a soft type of lactose sugar which is easily crushed into a powder. This melts rapidly in the mouth. Crush the tablets by using a clean dry spoon in a clean dry cup or bowl, or use a clean mortar and pestle.

The tiny #10 size pellets are satisfactory and may be placed between the infant's gum and cheek and allowed to dissolve there.

If your pellets are of a larger size, it is recommended that they be dissolved in water first, before being given to the infant. Bigger size pellets are not a problem with older children who are happy to dissolve the 'candy-like' pellets in their mouth.

In order that you may administer a remedy dissolved in water - four things are needed: a spoon, a glass, a saucer, and pure, filtered or distilled water.

1. First rinse the spoon, glass and saucer with pure water to remove any surface residues.

2. Add to the glass the equivalent of one dose of the remedy.

3. Half-fill the glass with pure water and stir thoroughly until dissolved. Note that if you forsee having to give the remedy a number of times, fill the glass half full. If you are anticipating giving the remedy only once or twice, fill the glass with less water, an ounce or two would be fine.

4. Stir the water until pellets/tablets are dissolved.

5. Using the spoon, place a little water inside the infant's mouth (1/4 tsp. is sufficient). If you cannot get the water on or under the tongue, it may be placed between the lip and the gum.

6. If you will be needing to give the remedy again within the next day or so, place the saucer on top of the glass and store it in a cool dark place away from strong odors. The remedy can thus be saved in liquid form for repeated doses over a period of several days.

Potency and Frequency of Usage for Infants

As a general rule it is recommended that lower potencies be given to infants. However, if the symptoms are intense, the remedy is clearly indicated, and the lower potency has helped but the effects are not lasting, then it is justified to give a higher potency, i.e., 30C. Follow the usage instructions given on your remedy vial or remedy kit brochure if available. Decrease frequency of use as infant improves and discontinue when improvement is well established.

Example:
Teething Infant with Diarrhea
Selected Remedy: Chamomilla 30C

Chamomilla 30C is first given in the early morning, with the infant clearly showing signs of improvement. The pain and irritability are lessened.

Chamomilla 30C is given a second time at noon. Improvement is continuing and the child seems much better. Stools are becoming more formed.

Later that afternoon the infant has another stool which looks almost normal.

By bedtime the child seems well but a third dose is then given. The child is 99% better and sleeps well.

The remedy would not be given on the following day if the baby was feeling 100% better.

However, if the infant still needed improvement, Chamomilla 30C could be repeated once that day to resolve the symptoms. Notice how the repetition has been reduced to reflect the improvement.

The frequency of usage depends on the situation and is not a mechanical process. These principles hold true for using homeopathy with all age groups.

READING ASSIGNMENT

Read pp. 150 - 157 in the TEXT up to Colic. As the remedies are discussed, turn to the chart pp. 163 - 170 and study the remedies there.
Note:
On p. 156, the TEXT defines Belladonna as a right sided remedy and indeed it is. However, if you have an earache case and all the symptoms match Belladonna and it is in the left ear, Belladonna could likely still be the remedy. So do not let 'sidedness' alone determine your decision. Remember the case analysis hint of prescribing *positively* based on the symptoms that *match* the remedy.

WRITTEN ASSIGNMENT

Find the remedy for each of the following cases based upon the TEXT, the Syllabus and BOERICKE. Referral back to Recommended Frequency of Usage on p. 16 of this Syllabus may be helpful.
Remember, case analysis for babies requires keen observation, as we cannot have a dialogue about the sensations of pain with an infant.

1. *Baby with Cold and suspected Earache*
(3) Thick and profuse light yellowish discharge from nose.
(2) Cough sounds loose, sound of mucus in chest.
The baby has been crying in an irritated way (1) and has sometimes been pulling at the ear (1).
(2) The baby's symptoms are improved in a warm environment.
Which remedy is closest?

Suppose you have the remedy in 12X potency and it is given three times the first day. Toward the evening, after the third dose the child is 20% better. The infant is 20% further improved the next morning. How often would you repeat the remedy on that day?

2. *Baby with Cold and suspected Earache*
(3) Thick and profuse light yellowish discharge from nose.
(2) Cough sounds loose; sounds of mucus in chest.
(2) The baby's symptoms are improved in open air.
(1) Baby has been crying for attention.
(1) Baby has occasionally been pulling at the ear.
What remedy is closest?

Note that the recommended repetition for 12C potency is two times a day. Suppose the remedy is given two times the first day and second day. On the third day the baby is 75% better and the dose is continued two times a day. On the fourth day the baby is 95% better. What repetition would you suggest for the fourth day and why?

3. *Name the three remedies that are known to develop a cold from exposure to cold. Which of those remedies matches this case?*

Baby with Cold:
The symptoms appeared suddenly (2) after exposure to cold (3). The baby is squirming about in bed (2). Her face is hot with one cheek red and the other cheek pale (3). The baby has a dry cough (2).
The baby received this remedy in 3C three times during the first six hours. But now she is 70% better. The symptoms are less intense. How often would you give the remedy now? Why?

4. *Baby with Earache*
Worse 9 p.m. - 11 p.m. (2). The baby is obviously in a lot of pain (3). She is crying furiously (3) and is thrashing about (3). She has been nursing more than usual (2). She seemed to be even worse after her grandmother turned up the heat (1). What is the remedy?

READING ASSIGNMENT

Read pp. 157 - 158. Colic in the TEXT. Read the colic remedies in the TEXT chart. Notice that Calcarea carbonica is another colic remedy, for colic due to milk intolerance. Read the supplementary colic remedies in the Syllabus.

Colic Differential

Magnesia carbonica / Mag. carb. / Mag-c.
Colicky pain with green diarrhea. Hates baby food made from vegetables.

Pulsatilla / Puls.
Indigestion. Whiny, moans a lot. Wants to nurse when sick. Indigestion etiology - eating ice cream.

Coffea cruda / Coff.
Colic with insomnia. Restlessness and sensitivity to noise and cold. Great sensitivity to pain.

READING ASSIGNMENT

Colocynthis Materia Medica.
Read Colocynthis in your remedy kit brochure if you have one. Then scan through Colocynthis in BOERICKE on pp. 227 - 228, placing emphasis on these sections: Abdomen and Modalities.
The remedy Colocynthis is the Bitter Cucumber, which has a high Phosphate of Magnesia content. Dr. Panos describes the remedy Magnesia Phosphorica in the TEXT materia medica which has an action that is quite similar to Colocynthis.

WRITTEN ASSIGNMENT

Colocynthis Materia Medica.
5. Colocynthis, known for its abdominal pains and cramps, causes the person to go into what position and do what to relieve the pain?

6. What emotional state could make Colocynthis pains worse?

READING ASSIGNMENT

Read pp. 159 - 161 in the TEXT, Diarrhea, Vomiting and Diaper Rash. As the remedies are discussed, look them up and study them in the chart on pp. 163 - 170.

Malabsorption Syndrome; Intolerance for Mother's Milk and Milk in General

The infant with this condition will characteristically have watery diarrhea after nursing, with vomiting of mother's milk. The abdomen may be distended. If not cared for, emaciation and dehydration develop.

Aethusa cynapium given as an acute before nursing may prevent the vomiting and enable the milk to be digested.

However, if the the symptoms persist when Aethusa is withdrawn, the infant needs a deeper remedy which should be prescribed by an experienced homeopathic physician. These deeper remedies could be Calcarea carbonica, Calcarea phosphorica, Silicea, Sulphur or Phosphorus, depending on the constitution of the child. Deeper constitutional treatment will be covered in more advanced courses.

READING ASSIGNMENT

Look up Aethusa cynapium in BOERICKE to see what it says about milk digestion.

READING ASSIGNMENT

Read pp. 161 - 162, Teething. As the teething remedies are discussed find and study them in the chart on pp. 163 - 170. Then study the supplementary Teething Differential which follows in the Syllabus.

In reviewing the truth that homeopathy acts by the law of similars, we must always find that remedy which specifically matches the symptoms. Dr. Panos has covered the prominent teething remedies. Here are some others which could be indicated.

Teething Differential

Coffea cruda / Coff.
Baby is in a wide awake, tense state, and is very sensitive. The nervous system is especially oversensitive to noises. The infant is in a lot of pain.

Phytolacca / Phyt.
The baby is clenching the jaws, and whatever teeth may be coming through, together. Baby is worse from warm drinks. Digging pains, if baby could talk to describe them.

Hepar sulph / Hep.
Mouth and gums are hypersensitive to touch. Pus or boils in gums with eruption of teeth. Silicea also has this.

Kreosotum / Kreos.
The teeth come in rotten, or when they erupt they show signs of decay. Dentition is painful and difficult. Restless sleep.

WRITTEN ASSIGNMENT

7. A baby is teething and has diarrhea. Based upon the following information find the remedy.

The baby wants things, but then refuses them or throws them away. Baby wants to be carried, then does not want to be carried. Nothing improves his mood.

8. A baby has an upset stomach with vomiting. Based upon the following information find the remedy.
The baby wants things, but then refuses them. She does not want to be moved or carried. Nothing soothes her. She is irritable.
You have the remedy in 6C potency; initially how often would you think to repeat it? After 40% improvement how often would you repeat the remedy?

9. A Colicky Infant with Diarrhea
I go to my neighbors' house to help them with their baby daughter's diarrhea. The following is observed:
The infant is curled up, with the hands pressed into the abdomen. The stools have a musty odor and look like jelly. What is the remedy?
Suppose it was given in 12X potency four times the first day with 80% improvement and three times the following day with total improvement. How often might the remedy be given on the third day?

READING ASSIGNMENT

Chamomilla Materia Medica
Read Chamomilla in the TEXT materia medica on p. 262 and, if available, in your remedy kit brochure.
Read Chamomilla in BOERICKE on pp. 187 - 198, scanning the material by placing emphasis on finding the same symptoms in the TEXT. Read the modalities carefully.

WRITTEN ASSIGNMENT

Chamomilla Materia Medica
10. Describe the mood of a Chamomilla child.

11. What is the threshold of pain tolerance in a Chamomilla case?

12. What temperature aggravates Chamomilla complaints?

13. Write the abbreviation for Chamomilla.

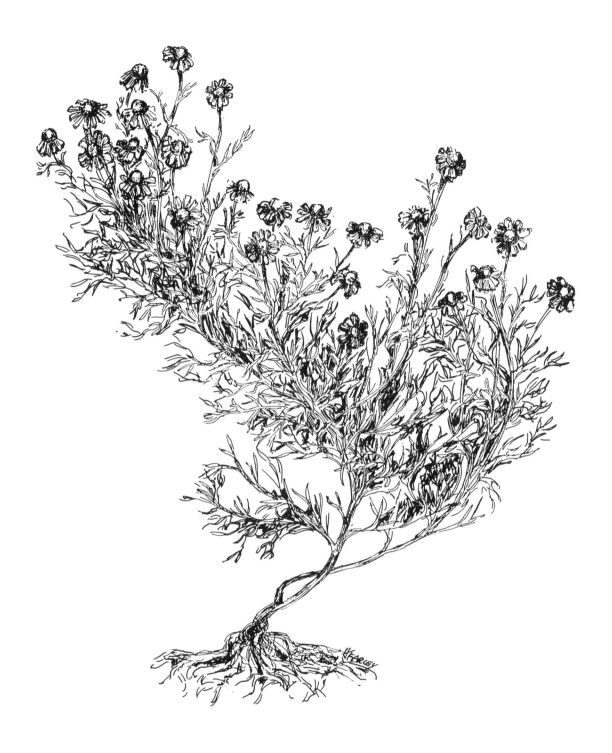

Chamomilla (German Chamomile)

* * * STOP * * *

Before you continue with the next lesson, send to your instructor your responses to all of the written assignments from Lessons 7 and 8. Any questions about the material covered thus far? Now is the time to send them in to your instructor.

Notes:

LESSON 9

Remedies for New-Borns

This information belongs to the realm of emergency health care. It is intended to be useful to know about - as a precautionary measure. This could be of use to those attending a home birth, and could be indispensable for midwives or health professionals delivering babies. If a situation should arise calling for one of these remedies, you are advised to give the correct remedy, clear the infant's air passageway, and seek emergency medical help. The correct remedy could make all the difference in the world.

<u>Cyanosis</u> - Babies born blue and not breathing properly

Laurocerasus / Laur.
Main remedy for babies who are born blue and not breathing.

Carbo veg. / Carb.-v.
The child is deathlike, ice cold, limp and blue. Carbo veg. is known as the 'corpse reviver.'

Veratrum album / Verat.
Beads of cold perspiration are on the forehead. Face is stoic and hard - similar to Carbo veg.

Antimonium tart. / Ant.-t.
Choking, gasping, drowning in own fluids. Deep globs of mucus in the chest. Known as the last gasp remedy, obstruction in respiratory tract. Deep rattle in chest - blue face.

Cuprum met. / Cupr.
Thumbs are clenched in and child is rigid. Not breathing due to spasm in bronchial tubes. Face and fingers blue. Thumbs are locked. No mucus in lungs, though.

Aconite / Acon.
Cyanosis - shock from the birth process. For fright of birth if other remedies do not act.

General Birth Trauma

Arnica / Arn.
Indicated if the birth process has been traumatic for the baby. The baby appears to have been bruised in the birth process. If the child is not pink and crying, clearly as a result of forceps delivery or birth trauma.

WRITTEN ASSIGNMENT

1. Find the remedy for this case:
Home Birth - Baby born blue.

The baby has a bluish coloration to the face and is struggling to breathe. It seems almost as though there is something obstructing the respiration. From time to time we hear the sound of loose fluid in the baby's lungs.
Find this remedy also under Colds in the TEXT and give the characteristics of the mucus in the chest with this remedy.

2. What remedy comes to mind for the baby who is born blue, when baby's hands are clenched in fists with the thumb clenched inside the fist? The baby is rigid as if in a spasm.

3. Home Birth: The birth process went fairly smoothly. However, the baby is born blue and not breathing. What is the remedy?

READING ASSIGNMENT

Antimonium tartaricum Materia Medica
Read Antimonium tart. in the TEXT materia medica on p. 257 and, if available, in your remedy kit brochure. Read Antimonium tart. in BOERICKE on pp. 58 - 60, scanning the material by placing emphasis on finding the same symptoms in the TEXT. Read the modalities carefully.

WRITTEN ASSIGNMENT

Antimonium tartaricum Materia Medica
4. Describe the cough of Antimonium tart., focusing on how it sounds and what happens with the mucus in the lungs.

5. Describe the energy of the Antimonium tart. case.

6. What temperature aggravates the symptoms?

7. Write the abbreviation for Antimonium tart.

The Growing Child

READING ASSIGNMENT

Read pp. 171 - 172 in the TEXT.

WRITTEN ASSIGNMENT

8. The experienced British homeopath, Dr. Gibson describes five remedies for poisoning. List each of these remedies and give a brief description differentiating the poisoning symptoms of each one.

READING ASSIGNMENT

Veratrum album Materia Medica
Read Veratrum album in the TEXT materia on p. 271 and, if available, in your remedy kit brochure. Read Veratrum album in BOERICKE on pp. 667 - 669, scanning the material by placing emphasis on finding the same symptoms in the TEXT. Read the modalities carefully.

WRITTEN ASSIGNMENT

Veratrum album Materia Medica
9. Describe the body temperature of a Veratrum alb. state.

10. Describe the perspiration in a Veratrum alb. state.

11. Describe the Veratrum alb. diarrhea state, giving the nature of the evacuation, the consistency, and the pains.

12. What temperature improves Veratrum album?

13. Write the abbreviation for Veratrum album.

READING ASSIGNMENT

Read pp. 173 - 179 in the TEXT, up to The School Age Child.

As a rule it is recommended to wait a minimum of 12 hours to assess the action of a remedy that has been given. For a child with a sore throat, therefore, we may give the remedy three to four times within a 12 hour period. We allow time to assess the results. If we were to be impatient we could possibly change the remedy shortly after giving the remedy the first time without allowing enough time to see the results. If there is no improvement after 12 hours, we are justified to change the remedy.

In the section on CROUP on p. 179, the TEXT mentions a well proven triad of remedies for this condition which has proven effective for over 150 years. If your child has croup, follow the method she describes on p. 179. Here the remedy is changed after an hour if there is no result, as one similarly might handle a painful earache. Of course, whenever there is severe breathing difficulty, emergency care is needed.

Caution: Do not let yourself get in the habit of changing remedies after an hour, routinely; in other acute conditions it can lead to confusion in one's case analysis and homeopathic work.

WRITTEN ASSIGNMENT

14. Describe the illness Croup. Include the main symptoms of the disease and the most common age groups of children affected.

15. What is the first remedy to be given at the onset of Croup?

16. What remedy is to be given after an hour from the first dose, if the symptoms persist?

17. If after the second hour the symptoms persist, with a hard and barking, ringing cough, what is the remedy to give?

READING ASSIGNMENT

Spongia tosta Materia Medica
Read Spongia tosta in the TEXT materia medica on p. 269 and, if available, in your remedy kit brochure. Read Spongia tosta in BOERICKE on pp. 603 - 604, scanning the material by placing emphasis on finding the same symptoms in the TEXT. Read the modalities carefully.

WRITTEN ASSIGNMENT

Spongia tosta Materia Medica
18. What atmospheric conditions can cause a Spongia cold?

19. Where does the Spongia cold usually begin?

20. Are the Spongia respiratory passages and cough wet and rattling with mucus or are they dry?

21. How can the voice be affected in a Spongia cold?

22. What temperature drinks improve the Spongia cold?

23. Around what time is Spongia worse?

24. What is the abbreviation for Spongia?

READING ASSIGNMENT

Read pp. 179 - 180 in the TEXT.

Nutritional guidelines for the child with recurring colds:

Serve less cheese and dairy products. Substitute soy products and sea vegetables for some of the dairy. Learn to prepare sea vegetables; they are high in calcium and minerals. Incorporate sprouts into the diet. Incorporate freshly extracted fruit and vegetable juices into the diet. Prepare snacking foods from nuts, seeds, and organic fruits and vegetables. Avoid processed denatured foods and foods with preservatives. Constitutional homeopathic treatment under the care of a homeopathic physician can eliminate the need for extremes in dietary limitations.

READING ASSIGNMENT

Read pp. 181 - 182, Tonsillitis in the TEXT. As you read each tonsillitis remedy, find it and study it in the chart on pp. 199 - 210. Consider the Sore Throat Differential in Lesson 5 as a supplement to the tonsillitis material given in this lesson.

WRITTEN ASSIGNMENT

NOTE: The TEXT and Syllabus differentials provide outstanding key note characteristics of the remedies as they apply to each illness. Life, however, is full of variety and complexity. When we see people in real life, the symptoms may not readily match the TEXT description, as we would like. Still, it may be that we are not looking thoroughly enough to find the symptoms. If the first remedy is not correct, it is necessary to look deeper at the symptoms.

25. Read the case of Tonsillitis which follows. In this case Mercurious was given and there are no signs of improvement whatsoever after 24 hours.

Case: Tonsillitis in a 5-year-old boy.
He is now complaining that his throat hurts (3). On looking at the throat we see the tonsils are red (3) and swollen (3). He feels worse and his throat hurts more during the hottest part of the day in the afternoon. His throat hurts more at night in sleep (2), especially if it is warm in bed (3). He has been having low energy and is irritable. He has not been thirsty (2) for anything except milk (2), which he has been drinking more of than usual.
Analyze this case. Write the symptoms in the proper format and write in the abbreviation of the remedy next to the symptoms each matches. In your analysis utilize the TEXT chart differential, mini-repertory and materia medica, the Syllabus differential and BOERICKE.

In your effort to solve this case you will be more successful by referring to the TEXT mini-repertory.
Referral to BOERICKE's materia medica at the completion of the analysis, to read about the remedy(ies) that figure strongly, will help you to decide.
Note: The remedy for this case is in most home remedy kits.

26. Analyze this case of Tonsillitis.
Write the symptoms out in the proper format with the corresponding remedy abbreviations next to them.
Refer to BOERICKE for your final decision. Try to find the symptom BASHFUL in BOERICKE, either in the Materia Medica by examining the remedies which seem close, or in the Repertory under Mind.

Tonsillitis - a girl four years old.
Tonsils are inflamed (3). She has had this several times in the past 6 months (1). The complaint seemed to start after being out on a cold winter day (2). There are sticking pains in the throat (1) which are worse from swallowing (1). The left tonsil is more inflamed (2). She feels worse if she lies on her left side (2). She has been acting especially bashful (3).

READING ASSIGNMENT

Ferrum phos Materia Medica.
Read Ferrum phos. in the TEXT materia medica on p. 262 and, if available, in your remedy kit brochure.
Note that on p. 263 of the TEXT there is an error. Ferrum phos. is WORSE 4 to 6 a.m. Go now to delete BETTER 4 to 6 a.m. from the TEXT and write in WORSE 4 to 6 a.m.
Read Ferrum phos. in BOERICKE on pp. 286 - 288, scanning the material by placing emphasis on finding the same symptoms found in the TEXT. Read the modalities carefully.

WRITTEN ASSIGNMENT

Ferrum phos Materia Medica.
27. List the complaints that Ferrum phos. is well known for treating.

28. For what stage in these illnesses is Ferrum phos. specifically indicated?

29. Describe the onset of a Ferrum phos. fever.

READING ASSIGNMENT

Read Childhood diseases in the TEXT pp. 182 - 183 up to Rubella. Add the following remedy in this Syllabus as a supplement to Measles.

Measles

Apis: A severe case. The rash has not come out yet and there is a puffy face with dry skin. The child is thirstless and may scream and cry. Apis brings out the rash and when the rash comes out there is relief.

WRITTEN ASSIGNMENT

30. Find the remedy for this early stage of Measles (7 day) based on the following symptoms:
Child is restless (2). Nose is running (2). Hard dry cough (1). Fever with chill (2). Face is pale (3), but cheeks have a rosy red coloration (3).

31. Find the remedy for this case of Measles (7 day) based on the following symptoms:
Eyes water (2). A lot of watery discharge coming from eyes (2). Eyelids stick together (2). The cough is dry (1) at night (1) but looser in the daytime (1). Feels worse in hot weather (2). Abundant thick yellow mucus (3) that is easily expectorated (3). Child desires attention and company (3).

READING ASSIGNMENT

Read pp. 183 Rubella through p. 186 (Scarlet Fever) in the TEXT.

WRITTEN ASSIGNMENT

32. What might a homeopathic physician give, as a preventative, to a pregnant woman who has not had Rubella and has been exposed to it?

33. Which Chicken Pox remedy has intense itching and restlessness and is aggravated by heat?

34. Which Chicken Pox remedy has intense itching, restlessness and is ameliorated by heat?

35. What remedy may be given to the adult who is exposed to Mumps who has not had Mumps, as a preventative?

36. Name the remedy which is specific for Scarlet Fever. Describe the classic picture of this remedy in Scarlet Fever.

37. What remedy may be taken as a Scarlet Fever preventative for someone who has been exposed to this disease?

READING ASSIGNMENT

Study pp. 187 - 189, Enuresis in the TEXT. As each remedy is discussed, find it and study it in the chart on pp. 199 - 214. Study the Enuresis supplementary differential in the Syllabus which follows.

In using homeopathy for Enuresis, it is recommended to give the remedy in 6C potency, three times a day. Allow two - four weeks for results. If the remedy selected does not work during/after this time, then you are justified to choose another remedy *if* it is clear to you. This means that there are definite symptoms which match the remedy you intend to give. Sometimes Enuresis is the sign of a deeper problem; such as diabetes, if there is frequent urination in large quantities, or it may also be an indication of a deep constitutional imbalance. In these cases see a homeopathic physician.

Enuresis (Bed Wetting) Differential

Causticum / Caust.
The Causticum child is more outgoing and sociable than the Sepia child. This is important to note, for these two remedies are difficult to distinguish in Enuresis. Causticum has loss of control of the bladder sphincter. This could arise from a situation where the child has to hold in urine for too long a time, e.g. A mean father on a car trip forces the child to hold it in, or in school the child is afraid to ask the teacher to let him go to the toilet. This leads to a loss of feeling in the urethra; no sensation of urination. Also can have retention of urine; takes a long time to urinate but urine passes when the eyes are closed.

Sepia / Sep.
Similar to Causticum. Sepia is a more withdrawn and shy child. Bedwetting occurs as soon as the child goes to sleep, within the first 1/2 hour, due to poor bladder sphincter tone. He may keep his mind on controlling it before going to sleep, but urine comes out when asleep. May also have dribbling of urine during laughter.

Equisetum / Equis.

Indicated where the child is healthy and has no other symptoms. Here bedwetting is out of habit only. Characteristically there is profuse pale urine with dreams and nightmares.

The recommended usage is three - five drops of Equisetum tincture in 1/2 glass of warm water three times a day, before meals.

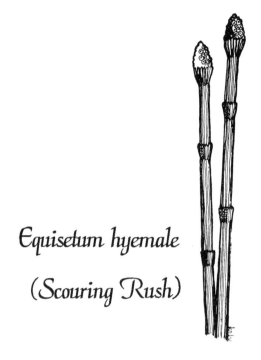

Equisetum hyemale

(Scouring Rush)

Lycopodium / Lyc.

Involuntary urination while asleep. There may be red sediment in the urine. Child wakes often to urinate. Child may be timid and shy and have poor confidence with a fear of failure and nervousness. There is often gas and bloating in the intestines. A mental/emotional etiology could be an aggressive father who makes the child tense. The child lets go and urinates in sleep. The father then becomes angry and punishes the child, who becomes even more tense - thus causing a vicious cycle.

Thuja

Has sudden urges to urinate and usually never makes it to the toilet - it is too late. Sometimes he may have to go six times in a night. The urine has a strong odor. Enuresis since vaccination, also could have warts and asthma. He may have sudden urges to urinate during the day and will grasp onto the parent until he gets to the bathroom.

Phosphorus / Phos.

Enuresis related to too much thirst. Excessive drinking of cold drinks - there is a craving for ice water. Phosphorus usually suits more of a tall slender type of child who is sensitive to impressions and is sympathetic.

Benzoic acid / Benz-ac.

The outstanding characteristic of this Enuresis is that the urine is dark colored and has a strong ammoniacal odor that permeates everything. Urine stains the sheets brown.

Arsenicum album / Ars.

Enuresis related to insecurity, anxiety, and nervousness.

WRITTEN ASSIGNMENT

*38. Jonah, a boy seven years old, has always had Enuresis. It used to be worse, now he wets the bed about twice a week. Aside from this problem, his family doctor says he is in excellent health and has no other health complaints. His parents, strict adherents to holistic health, have refused vaccinations for him. Jonah was born at home and has never been to a hospital His urine does not smell especially strong and does not leave stains in the bedding.
What remedy would you choose for this case?*

*39. Lisa, a girl six years old, has been having problems with Enuresis ever since she had to hold it in during a long bus ride going to summer camp. Her mother can provide no other symptoms except that she wets her bed just after falling asleep. We notice that she made friends with other people in the waiting room and is sociable.
What remedy would you choose for this case?*

40. Which remedy might you select for the above case if Lisa was a shy withdrawn type of child?

*41. Timothy is eight and recently developed Enuresis when his parents divorced. He had to move out-of-state with his mother. Having left his father, familiar friends, and accustomed surroundings, he feels insecure and afraid. He seem to be more chilly than usual, and we notice he is restless.
What remedy might we select for Timothy's condition?*

LESSON 10

WRITTEN ASSIGNMENT

Paper Case
This is your only written assignment for Lesson 10. Send in to your instructor one acute case which you have taken, recorded, and analyzed. Note that an acute case involves an ailment of temporary duration of less that three weeks which can be treated at home with self-care.*

Certainly by now you have encountered a common acute ailment out of the many possible ailments mentioned in the TEXT, Homeopathic Medicine at Home. *So, don't hesitate - simply present one case you have taken. Be sure to check the organization of your case data and the analysis so that it is as complete as possible.*

You will receive guidance in your development of skills in casetaking, organization of case data and in case analysis. This paper case is for learning purposes only and must not be construed as prescribing on the part of your instructor.

*A complaint which has been in existence for a month or more is usually considered to be chronic. Chronic complaints require a deep constitutional homeopathic treatment and should be brought to the attention of your homeopathic physician.

READING ASSIGNMENT

Read pp. 189 - 190 in the TEXT, Fears and Anxieties.

In case analysis of a child, our observations of the child's personality or mood can be a deciding factor in the selection of a remedy. Observation of the child's personality and energy state is especially important when using homeopathy for symptoms such as fears.

The following Child's Eye Differential represents an immensely practical collection of the characteristics observed in children as they apply to the homeopathic remedies. Be sure to refer to this material when using homeopathy for an emotional state in a child or when some aspect of the child's mood is outstanding. Also included in the differential are some valuable aspects of the remedies relating to etiology and physical traits.

This Child's Eye Differential serves as an introduction to the sphere of action of the homeopathic remedies on a personality level. This aspect of homeopathy is fascinating and it can be quite effective in balancing the personality. The personality level represents the deepest part of the being in the hierarchy of health. Only after a training in advanced constitutional homeopathy is one qualified to use homeopathy for deep imbalances. The beginning student of homeopathy is advised to leave case analysis of deep personality imbalances to a homeopathic physician.

It is simpler to begin one's study of the personality aspects of the remedies as they relate to children. This is so because children have been through fewer experiences, and it is easier to discern the remedy images in them. Adults often have been through numerous tribulations which can cause the original personality pattern to change. In adults there may be several layers that need treatment before one gets back to the original state. This belongs to the sphere of advanced homeopathy. It is worthwhile to note, however, that these personality essences as they relate to children can also be translated to relate to adults. Within each remedy there will be a similarity between the personality pattern of the adult state and the child state.

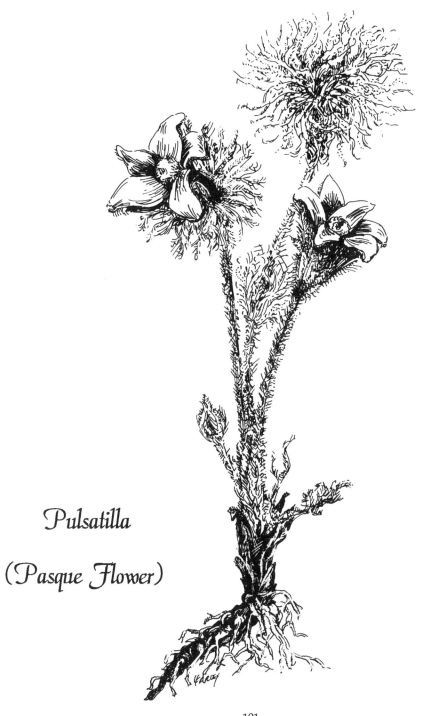

Pulsatilla

(Pasque Flower)

Read the following Child's Eye Differential. Read each remedy in an unhurried way, one at a time. With each one try to visualize the image of the child that is described. And try to think of one child you have met who matches this image. This will enable it to make an impression on your memory and you will be better equipped to recognize it in real life.

Child's Eyes Differential

Pulsatilla / Puls.

Pitifulness. The eyes cry out for something and say - pity me. There is a sense of helplessness and loneliness. These children have a very strong desire for love and attention. They may act as if they cannot do things to get more attention. Observing the child evokes a mothering instinct. It is as if the child goes through a biological change to make herself look pitiful and huggable. The eyes are big and pitiful, they pull at you and say - hug me. A very dependent child. In a shopping mall this child will be by the mother, making faces or flirting with people. Wants hurt kissed. Gets physiological relief from affection. If jealous will go to her room and talk to doll.

Pulsatilla Etiologies:

Child was strong and independent, and mother went back to work too soon - child felt abandoned. Child weaned too soon; mother goes away. Independent child gets sick and slips into a babyish state.

Tuberculinum / Tub.

Anger, menace in their eyes. There is a mean intent, a focused look. Looks right at you with piercing eyes. The eyes of an adult inside a little child. Has a desire to break things. The whole body tightens when angry. Hyperactive. Malicious, restless children with an inexhaustible energy. Gets in fights with other children. Pinches other child. If jealous, is mean and wants to get back. Has a very expressive earthy intensity. There is a tendency to have sore throats, tonsillitis, and upper respiratory infections. Desires cold milk and smoked meats, if exposed to them, and has a big appetite.

Arsenicum album / Ars.

Clinging, insecure, dependent eyes. Clinging to the mother like a baby monkey. There is fear in his eyes. He is in a frightening place and needs protection. The child may cry and scream when the mother leaves him off at the nursery school in the morning. In a shopping mall the child's eyes would show fright and he would be clinging to the mother. The child is chilly and thirsty for sips.

Baryta carbonica / Bar-c.

There is a sense of dumb wonderment in the eyes of these children. They do not understand or comprehend what is going on. They could be mentally retarded, but they do not have to be. In an educational setting the teacher would see the child trying hard to understand, but there would be an incomprehension with a sense of wonderment.

Baryta carb. Etiologies:

Child is deprived of something, e.g., is left at home or gets frightened when having a serious illness. Something gets altered in the child's stability.

Natrum muriaticum / Natrum mur. / Nat.-m.

These children look away if you look in their eyes. There is emotional sensitivity in their eyes. They have an eagerness to anticipate doing the right thing. They do as the parents wish. Not fussy children. They do not want to be rejected. It hurts Natrum mur. children to be stared at; they could break out crying in this situation. Typically the eyes of these children are oversensitive to the sun. These children, in contrast to the affectionate Pulsatilla children, could have an aversion to being touched. Child is more introverted emotionally. Desires salty foods.

Phosphorus / Phos.

There is a twinkle in their eyes. The eyes are happy, with a look of excitement and aliveness. The eyes can seem a little spacey and are not focused. These children dislike being alone. They have a fear of thunderstorms. Expressive, sociable children. Desire for cold drinks, and salty foods.

Sulphur / Sulph.

Has the intent of Tuberculinum eyes but the excitement of Phosphorus eyes. Piercing eyes, with an investigative excitement. Piercing lively, imaginative, children. When playing with other children Sulphur would be the leader of the group. They can be inquisitive, curious children who are very adept and coordinated physically. Can also be children of intellectual parents with a lopsided overdevelopment of the mind. Absorbed in comic books. These children enjoy taking things apart; they have a desire to fix things. They have an aversion to bathing, especially the head.

Lycopodium / Lyc.

These children have shaky, self-conscious eyes. They are always anticipating what they are doing and how they look. They have a fear of failing and making mistakes. There is a sense of shyness, yet they tend to arrogant with younger children.
Lycopodium Etiologies:
Domineering mother and father make child nervous and uptight. Child has unusual physical features, e.g., big ears, and is made fun of in school. Child in school with foreign accent, is made fun of.

Silicea / Sil.

Their eyes show a deep fragility. They are like little glass dolls which say - do not bump me or make me do anything strenuous. These children are very delicate and weak and are not tough like other children. They can get injured or short of breath easily. Thin, emaciated children with a tendency to respiratory problems. The complexion may be pale.
Silicea Etiologies:
Prematurely born babies. Nursing from an undernourished mother. Vaccinations leading to recurring illnesses treated with antibiotics, causing the child to be weaker and lose weight.

Calcarea carbonica / Calcarea carb. / Calc.

Sluggish physical makeup, delayed dentition. Suits a large percentage of children up to age two and a half years. They are like mini-adults, imitating and copying adults. Very orderly children. They have a natural helping instinct. These children can have cold wet feet. Can have a calcium imbalance. In a shopping mall these children are investigative. They are independent children.

Staphysagria / Staph.

The eyes talk to you and it is a message of apology and fear. These children are timid and mild. Their eyes say 'I apologize, it's my fault.'
Staphysagria Etiology:
The child who is sexually abused by the parent.

Stramonium / Stram.
The eyes have the look of a wild animal. They are fixed, wide open, and sparkling. Often associated with high fevers or mental derangement.

Belladonna / Bell.
The eyes look wild; associated with high fever and delirium. The pupils are enlarged. There is inquietude and restlessness. The child is flushed and hot.

Causticum / Caust.
The eyes are quite similar to Phosphorus. They are excitable, affectionate, and outgoing. They are sensitive children who are very perceptive and are easily connected with their environment. Their sensitivity makes them susceptible to fright and grief and they may develop twitches. Also sensitive to cold dry winds.

Case Analysis of Children's Mental / Emotional States

When selecting a homeopathic remedy for a child's mental/emotional state, we consider the mental/emotional state as the Chief Complaint, the most important symptom. In our analysis we look to see if there is an etiology or causative situation for the problem. In the TEXT example on p. 190, disappointment was the etiology for the despondency in the Ignatia case.

We also examine the child's General Symptoms, such as body temperature, thirst, perspiration, general appearance and energy. When analyzing a mental/emotional state in a child, we also consider dietary cravings or aversions.

The three factors to consider in analyzing children's Mental/Emotional states are:
1. Chief Complaint - Child's Mental/Emotional state.
2. Etiology
3. General Symptoms.

In previous lessons we have not emphasized dietary cravings/aversions as characteristics of the child because they are not necessary considerations and could become confusing in the acute case analysis we are learning. When analyzing fears, however, some remedies have outstanding dietary characteristics, which help to decide the remedy.

Frequency of Usage and Potency for Mental / Emotional Complaints in Adults and Children

In using homeopathy for mental/emotional states the recommended frequency of usage for beginners is two doses of 30C potency: one in the AM and one in the PM on a single day. **That is for one day only.** (Before giving the remedy, carefully study the symptoms to be sure they match the remedy). Then one waits a month to see the results. If after a month the adult or child is improved, then one waits as long as the improvement lasts. Only if the improvement relapses does one consider employing homeopathy again.

If the improvement relapses or there is no improvement this is an indication of a deeper imbalance and you are advised to consult a homeopathic physician. It is an undesirable situation to be giving homeopathic remedies without knowing what is happening, in a guessing way. Do not allow yourself to fall into this situation. This is especially important with potencies of 30C and higher. Follow the advice of the TEXT in Beyond First Aid on p. 190.

Child's Fear Differential

FEAR OF MONSTERS

Calcarea carbonica / Calc.

They have strong imaginations and may actually see the monster. Can have nightmares of monsters and wake screaming. These children are sensitive to people or animals in trouble. They tend to be overweight, soft, and in some cases, chilly. In other cases Calcarea carbonica children have good body warmth. They perspire on the head during sleep. They crave eggs, sweets, and sometimes dairy products.

Phosphorus / Phos.

These children are sensitive to impressions. They might believe a ghost story and, with their strong impressionable imagination, see the phantom. They are sympathetic, sociable children known to be afraid of thunderstorms. They tend to be tall and slender in build and they desire cold drinks. Predisposition to colds and bronchial affections.

Note: Both Calcarea carb. and Phosphorus children have similarities in their fears. it is helpful to examine the General Symptoms of the child in order to decide on the remedy.

Lycopodium / Lyc.

These children can often be observed to breathe through their mouths during sleep. A tendency to wrinkle the forehead may also be seen. Excessive intestinal gas or general predisposition to digestive upsets may be present. As a rule, they prefer warm foods and drinks instead of cold. They crave sweets.[1]

Stramonium / Stram.

Actually see the monster and have terrible nightmares of witches and demons. They may freak out and scream in terror. Faces come at them. This phenomenon may come on during a fever or delirium. Have to have the lights on at night.

FEAR OF THE DARK

Calcarea carbonica / Calc.
Imagines something is there - worries.

Phosphorus / Phos.
Also imagines something is there, but is more impressionable that Calcarea carb.

Stramonium / Stram.
Fear of the dark during a fever or delirium. Has to have the lights on.

Pulsatilla / Puls.
Fear of being alone in the dark. Pulsatilla is afraid of being alone and desires company.

Arsenicum album / Ars.
Frightens very easily. The dark gives the child a feeling of being unable to breathe or gives a feeling that no one will come to help him. Tosses and turns in sleep. Deeply restless. Could have respiratory problems. Chilly, sensitive to cold, and thirsty for sips.

---

[1]Practically all children have a desire for sweets. The fact that a child has this trait, in itself, is not sufficient information for basing a remedy selection.

FEAR AT MOVIES

Calcarea carbonica / Calc.
Sensitive and impressionable. Examine the General Symptoms to decide.

Phosphorus / Phos.
Sensitive to impressions and gullable. They can feel the characters in the movie as if they themselves were experiencing it.

Causticum / Caust.
These children are excitable, perceptive, and very sensitive. They are interested in what is going on in their surrounding environment. They feel worse in cold dry winds and crave smoked or spicy foods.

FEAR SOMETHING IS GOING TO HAPPEN TO PARENTS

Pulsatilla / Puls.
An affectionate child who is very attached to the parents, especially the mother. The Pulsatilla child can have a fear of being abandoned or being alone. He can have nightmares of the parents going away.

Arsenicum album / Ars.
Arsenicum children are very attached to the parents. They are nervous and restless. Desirous of warmth and thirsty for sips often, they are insecure and very fearful.

Calcarea carbonica / Calc.
These children can worry a lot. Look for other Calc. carb. symptoms.

Phosphorus / Phos.
These children are impressionable. For example, she sees a program on TV and becomes afraid that this could happen to her parents.

FEAR OF DOGS

The following remedies are known for the fear of dogs in children. To choose the correct remedy:
Take the child's case. Refer to the Child's Eye Differential in your analysis for matching the personality picture. Then look to match other General Symptoms in the TEXT. By looking up the remedies which appear close in BOERICKE, you should be able to find the remedy which best matches the symptoms.

- Tuberculinum
- Calcarea carb.
- Causticum
- Stramonium
- Belladonna.

* * * STOP * * *

Before you continue with the next lesson, send to your instructor your responses to all of the written assignments from Lesson 9 and 10. If you have any further questions about the material covered thus far, now is the time to send them in to your instructor.

Notes:

LESSON 11

Review of Case Analysis
for Children

WRITTEN ASSIGNMENT

Find the remedy for each of the following cases. Write the abbreviation of the remedies next to the symptoms they match, if you need to.

1. *A boy five years old with fear of dogs.*

Desires cold milk (3) and bacon (3). He is always on the go,.. - moving around (1), and has an intense energy (2). He has a very strong will power (2) and will become mean and will break things when angry (3).

2. *A girl five years old with fear of dogs.*

She is a little overweight, and physically slow (3). She is also afraid of the dark (1), and desires eggs (2). She is a chilly little person (3).

3. *Maria is affectionate (1) and sociable (3). She prefers to be with people (2) and is sensitive to any impressions. She gets startled easily from thunderstorms (2) and sonic booms (3). She loves potato chips (2) and spring water (2).*
Which remedy best matches her personality and the General Symptoms given?

4. *John, age 10, is a somewhat shy (2), introverted child. He seems to be self-conscious (3) and does not have many friends. He was born with slightly crossed eyes and is very self conscious about it. He plays with younger kids and is authoritarian and bossy with them (3).*
Which remedy best matches John's personality?

5. *John's seven-year-old brother Sam is outgoing (3). He loves to play chess on his computer (2) and has good concentration. When with his friends, he likes to determine what they will play (2). His eyes are focused (3), but not malicious.*
Which remedy best matches Sam's personality?

6. *Kenneth's father took him to see a scary movie with extraterrestrials. Ever since the movie he is afraid of the dark (3). He is afraid an extraterrestrial is there (3). Kenneth is compassionate with other children (1) and he likes cold drinks.*
Which remedy best matches Kenneth's personality, and General Symptom?

7. Sara, age 8, is staying with her aunt for two weeks while her parents take a cruise to Jamaica. Sara has expressed to her aunt an apprehension about something happening to her parents (3). She is of medium build and is not quick physically (3). Her aunt has been serving her favorite things: omelets and sweets (2). Her perspiration during sleep wets the pillow (3).
Which remedy fits Sara the best?

8. Tina, age five, is afraid of being alone (3). She is an affectionate (2) little girl and likes to stay up at night when her parents have company, to be the center of attention (2). Tina does not like to have to go to sleep alone. She cries easily (2) and requires a lot of affection (3) from her family.
Which remedy best suits Tina?

Adolescents and Young Adults

READING ASSIGNMENT

Read pp. 190 - 192 in the TEXT through Menstruation and study the remedies discussed in the Chart on pp. 199 - 215.

NOTE: The TEXT mentions Magnesia phos./Mag phos. as a remedy for menstrual cramps. The remedy Colocynthis is quite similar to Magnesia phos. The menstrual cramps of both remedies are relieved by warmth. Both remedies are relieved by bending double and applying pressure. Compare the Female, Abdomen, and Modalities heading for these two remedies in BOERICKE.

This similarity likely exists because the plant Colocynthis (Bitter Cucumber) contains Magnesia phos. as part of its chemical makeup - an interesting observation. Usually you will be successful in substituting these remedies. However, in cases where abdominal cramping is aggravated or caused by anger or indignation, Colocynthis would be a better choice.

WRITTEN ASSIGNMENT

9. In cases of severe Magnesia phos. menstrual pain, what method does the TEXT provide for taking the remedy?
Why might this method not be advisable for an Apis menstrual cramp? (If you are not sure, check in the TEXT materia medica.)

10. Which remedy seems best indicated for the menstrual cramps in this teenage girl?
She complains of pulsating pains (3), which come suddenly with intensity (3) and then they are not so bad for awhile. She describes a feeling as if the female organs are pushing down (1). The menstrual flow is bright red (2). She has a fever and her eyes are sensitive to light (2).

11. Which menstrual colic remedy would come to mind in the case of a teenager who is very irritable (3) and has severe pains which seem intolerable (3)?
Based on the above information, how would you suppose this girl would be affected by warm applications over the region of her uterus? (Check the TEXT materia medica if you are uncertain.)

Read pp. 192 - 196 to Mononucleosis in the TEXT. Find Kali Bromatum in BOERICKE and read the skin heading.

NOTE: The use of oral contraceptives either for birth control or controlling acne can interfere with the hormonal balance of the body. Hormonal imbalances once created can be difficult to resolve, even with the most astute homeopathic care.

WRITTEN ASSIGNMENT

12. Relating to the Law of Direction of Cure, how does a homeopath generally feel about treating skin ailments?

Poison Ivy / Poison Oak

A correctly chosen remedy will often relieve the intense discomfort and rapidly promote healing of poison ivy or poison oak. The following remedies are those most commonly recommended. However, it is still possible that the correct remedy could be one not listed in the differential which follows. If you are under the care of a homeopath, it is a good idea to obtain his or her approval before performing homeopathic self-care, especially in the case of skin complaints.

Anacardium / Anac.
Typically has intensely itching vesicular (blister-like) eruptions. They could also be burning. The main keynote to remember is that the itching is *made worse* from warm or hot water, or applications.

Rhus toxicodendron / Rhus tox.
Typically has intense burning-itching vesicular (blister-like) eruptions. Touch aggravates the itching. Opposite to Anacardium, Rhus tox. is *improved* by warm or hot water or applications.

Croton tig.
Has vesicular eruptions most commonly located on the genitals, scalp, and around the eyes. The sensations on the skin can be those of itching followed by burning. The skin can feel 'hide bound' or tight. Either a slight rubbing will relieve the itching or the person cannot bear to scratch hard because it hurts.

Grindelia Lotion [1]
Recommended for external application to relieve itching, burning vesicular eruptions.

Graphites / Graph.
Can be useful in later or more advanced stages where there are thick, oozing, crusty scabs discharging a sticky honey-like fluid. The crusts may appear more at the bends of limbs, i.e., elbow. The crusts can have deep cracks in them where the limb has been bent. Itching and burning sensations are common. The itching would tend to be worse from warmth, especially in a warm bed at night.

---

[1]Grindelia is available from homeopathic pharmacies as a tincture. To prepare Grindelia into a lotion follow the recommended procedure for making tinctures into lotions on p. 17 Syllabus.

READING ASSIGNMENT

Read pp. 196 - 197 to Emotions.

Note: Another remedy to consider for Mononucleosis is Gelsemium. Consider Gelsemium if Cistus does not act or the symptoms match Gelsemium better. Read the descriptions in BOERICKE before making your decision.

Gelsemium Mononucleosis:
The eyelids are heavy and there is dullness of mind with a feeling of malaise, and weakness. The person is apathetic and 'wiped out.' With the dullness of mind there is an internal feeling of trembling.

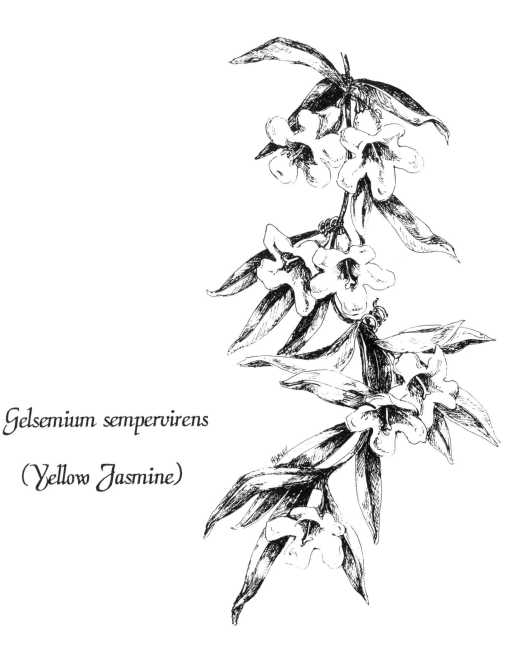

Gelsemium sempervirens

(Yellow Jasmine)

WRITTEN ASSIGNMENT

Gelsemium Mononucleosis:
13. *What season and weather are most conducive for Gelsemium colds and flu?*

14. *Describe the onset of Gelsemium.*

15. *Situations causing emotional stress can lead to physical ailments which correspond to Gelsemium. Give two examples of typical life situations which could cause a Gelsemium state. (Refer to BOERICKE).*

16. *How would you characterize the general energy and state of mind of the Gelsemium person?*

17. *Write the abbreviation for Gelsemium.*

READING ASSIGNMENT

Gelsemium Materia Medica
Read Gelsemium in the TEXT materia medica on p. 263 and, if available, in your remedy kit brochure. Read Gelsemium in BOERICKE on pp. 299 - 302, scanning the material by placing emphasis on finding the same symptoms in the TEXT. Read the modalities carefully.

Emotional Complaints

READING ASSIGNMENT

Read pp. 197 - 198, Emotions, in the TEXT.

Homeopathy has a significant sphere of action on mental/emotional complaints. It is a pity that the majority of the general public in the United States are unaware of this. The TEXT has done a great service by pointing out the side effects of conventional medicines. Why should people resort to drugs for mental/emotional complaints, when properly administered homeopathic remedies work so quickly and powerfully? The homeopathic remedy actually strengthens and stimulates the energy and personality of the person. The same cannot be said for conventional medicine.

Both Ignatia and Natrum mur. are remedies for grief and disappointing situations. There is a similarity between these two remedies, and they are known as complementary remedies. Complementary remedies in homeopathy, as the name implies, are remedies whose actions have a close and harmonious relationship. Look now on p. 42 in the very back of BOERICKE[1] Relationship of Remedies Chart, at Ignatia and see Ntr. M. - Natrum mur., as the complement. Information on the relationships between remedies may also be found under the individual remedies listed in BOERICKE. For example see p. 344 BOERICKE - Ignatia - Relationship - Complementary: Nat. mur.

For grief and disappointment, Ignatia is usually given first and has a beneficial effect. Sometimes it is all that is necessary. Where the grief is of long standing, Natrum mur. might be required and it is commonly one of the remedies given after Ignatia.

Ignatia amara/Ignatia Personality Picture

Ignatia is specific for a death in the family, a broken love relationship or other shocking, disappointing event. The sooner it is given, the better it is for the person. In the early stages of upset the person may cry easily, and be hysterical or moody.

Ignatia is also indicated for conflicts and anger in relationships.

Note: In order to give a person Ignatia for grief - anger and conflict do not *have* to be present.

Where there is a pattern of conflict, think of Ignatia. A teenager may be in conflict with his parents. His values may be different and there may be arguing and conflict at home. He may want to leave home, while being equally attached to the love and security of his family; conflict again. A divorce could be an example of conflict calling for Ignatia. Naturally with this kind of conflict there is anger.

The Ignatia type of person is perfectionistic and idealistic. Ignatia can also be critical, argumentative and irritable. Because they have such high ideals these people are especially subject to disappointments and grief from our apparently imperfect existence. They tend to hold a lot of tension. Ignatia is characteristically chilly and cannot tolerate cigarette smoke. Typically the Ignatia person will sigh when being questioned. So the homeopath needs to be on his or her toes to look for the sighs.

READING ASSIGNMENT

Ignatia amara Materia Medica
Read Ignatia amara (Ignatia) in the TEXT materia medica on p. 264 and, if available, in your remedy kit brochure. Read Ignatia in BOERICKE on pp.. 342 - 344, scanning the material by placing emphasis on finding the same symptoms noted in the preceding paragraph in the Syllabus and the TEXT.

---

[1]In some non-Indian editions of BOERICKE, the Relationship of Remedies Chart may be missing. In this case find this information under the individual remedy listed as in the above example of Ignatia on p. 344.

Ignatia amara Materia Medica
18. How would cigarette smoke and coffee tend to affect an Ignatia person?

19. List three life circumstances which could put a person into an Ignatia state.

Natrum muriaticum / Natrum mur. Personality Picture

The remedy Natrum mur. is derived from sea salt. In the event of grief or disappointment, Natrum mur. is to be thought of where the event has long since past and the person remains affected. This would be especially true in situations where either Ignatia was given and some symptoms matching Natrum mur. remain, or where Ignatia was never given. Ignatia and Natrum mur. are complementary. It is common for Natrum mur. to follow Ignatia, however depending on the case there are many other possible remedies which might follow Ignatia.

The Natrum mur. person will be more settled into his grief. He is weighed down by it and may be depressed. Always his mind will look back to unhappy past events. A Natrum mur. person would be less expressive emotionally. He would not like to have someone try to console him and prefers to be alone. Typically, the eyes are sensitive to the sun. It is common for the Natrum mur. type to desire salty foods and have great thirst. Lips may be dry and cracked.

Nux vomica/Nux.-v. Personality Picture

There is a similarity between Ignatia and Nux vomica. Both remedies contain the poison, strychnine. To remind you, this is absolutely harmless and of great benefit, in homeopathic form.

If the anger is not coming from a conflict and is quite evident, consider Nux vomica. The Nux vomica anger and irritability could be said to be more volatile that the Ignatia anger. Competitive, ambitious people who are likely to develop gastric disturbances. Desires alcohol, coffee, and spicy foods. In the adult, Nux vomica would be the pressured business executive who is competitive, aggressive and takes the above mentioned foods.

WRITTEN ASSIGNMENT

Note: Before completing written assignments 20 - 23, review **Frequency of Usage and Potency for Mental/Emotional Complaints for Adults and Children** p. 104 Syllabus.

20. Anton is sixteen years old. His parents want him to continue studying violin, but he instead wants to take up fencing. Neither side will give in. Anton also would like more freedom in the evenings to go out with this friends. Again here his parents oppose him. As a result of these conflicts Anton is irritable (3) and argumentative (3). The stress is showing in hypersensitivity to his father's cigars.
What remedy would you think to give Anton and in what potency and frequency of usage?

21. *Usha is a mild natured person. A dear friend of hers recently passed on and this was a shock to her. She has been crying a lot (3).*
What remedy would you consider for her grief?

22. *Martine is 15 years old. Her mother is worried because she has not started to menstruate regularly (2). Her moods are erratic (2). She can be laughing at one moment and the next moment be crying. She is affectionate (3) and because of this her mother is concerned about Martine getting prematurely involved in a relationship. Martine loves nature (2) and open air (2).*
Which remedy would you give Martine and in what potency and frequency of usage? How long would you wait to see the results? What would you do if the remedy did not act?

23. *Jay is a high school student. Last year, in the same month, his best friend died in a car accident, and he was not accepted for his desired position on the football team. He has not gotten over these griefs.*
He is keeping to himself often (2) and thinks of the past (2).
What remedy would you think to give Jay and in what potency and frequency of usage? How long would you wait to see the results? What would you do if the remedy did not act?

LESSON 12

Women's Health

READING ASSIGNMENT

Read pp. 216 - 219 up to Pregnancy in the TEXT. Examine each of the Headache remedies in the chart pp. 230 - 240. Be sure to read the Specific Headache Indications, the General Symptoms and Modalities for each remedy.

WRITTEN ASSIGNMENT

Find the remedies for the following two cases. Use the TEXT and BOERICKE for your analysis. Include with your answer a written copy of your analysis in the proper format.

1. Case: Headache with Diarrhea
Note: In this case the Chief Complaint is the headache. However, in this case, you might not be able to find the matching remedies for the headache symptoms. By reviewing the advice given for analysis of coughs in Lesson 6, p. 63 of this Syllabus, your analysis will be facilitated.

Mira is complaining of a headache (2) with diarrhea (1). Tomorrow she is scheduled to give a lecture for a large audience, upon which her career hinges. She seems shaky (2) and weak (2). She describes her whole head as feeling dull, heavy and (2) aching. Upon inquiring about the appearance of the diarrhea, she seems embarrassed but manages to say it is light colored (1). Mira's tongue is coated yellow (3). She has low energy (2) and seems a little better out-of-doors (1).

2. Case. Headache with Nausea.
Note: In solving this case take special care first to identify the Chief Complaint.

John's whole head feels as if it has a pressing pain (1). The pain feels better when he is resting quietly (1). His headache is also worse in the sun (2), from any noise (2), and from touching the head (2). He feels chilly. He is nauseous, but cannot vomit (3). He wants the interview to finish soon so he can go back to the football game on TV (2).

READING ASSIGNMENT

Read Pregnancy and Morning Sickness in the TEXT, pp. 219 - 220. As the remedies are discussed examine them in the chart on pp. 230 - 240. Study the Morning Sickness Differential which follows in the Syllabus.

Morning Sickness Differential

Colchicum / Colch.
Very sensitive to the smell of food and cooking.

Ipecac / Ip.
Indicated for severe morning sickness. There is nausea all the time and nothing relieves it. The stomach hangs down with a sinking feeling. This dragging sensation in the stomach is worse before and after eating. There is a disgust for food and drink. Ipecac has symptoms and modalities which are similar to Pulsatilla, namely, thirstless, worse warm stuffy rooms, worse fatty food. But Ipecac is more severe that Pulsatilla. Do you remember the appearance of the tongue in Ipecac?

Ignatia / Ign.
Pregnancy is not what it was expected to be - the woman had a false idea of pregnancy and learns it is hard work and it is not all a bed of roses. She is impatient, irritable, on edge, and very sensitive. There may be general hysteria. The stomach is knotted up with cramps.

Sepia / Sep.
The thought of food sickens. There is a bitter taste in the mouth, with severe nausea. May have delusions of smells that are not there. Other symptoms can be severe constipation, and depression with irritability. She will yell at her children.

Pulsatilla / Puls.
She presents a picture of helplessness and cries easily. She has capricious food cravings and does not really know what she wants. There is indigestion, nausea, with thirstlessness, and aggravation from fatty foods and warm stuffy rooms, as with Ipecac.

Nux vomica / Nux.-v.
She has retching with abdominal cramps in the morning until the mid-afternoon, when it goes away. She has nausea similar to a hangover, and has a toxic sluggish quality. She is irritable.

Anacardium / Anac.
Her nausea is improved while she is eating. About two hours after eating she becomes nauseous again. She has an empty feeling in the stomach and is always snacking. She has indigestion, gas and bloating. Wakes from sleep unrefreshed.

Cocculus / Cocc.
She has dizziness from motion, riding in train, car or bus, worse while reading. Can cause loss of sleep and lead to miscarriage. She is drained, weak, and dizzy.

Natrum muriaticum / Nat.-m.
Morning sickness with headaches that last all day. She is worse in the sun, withdrawn and depressed.

WRITTEN ASSIGNMENT

3. Stephanie is two months pregnant and has been having morning sickness for the past few weeks. The smell of food or even the thought of it makes her nauseous (3). She has an aversion to food (3).
What remedy would you give Stephanie?

4. Sandra is one and a half months pregnant and has developed morning sickness. The smell of food or even the thought of it makes her nauseous (3). She has been more irritable (3) than usual and had an imaginary smell of frankfurters in her kitchen which made her nauseous (3).
What remedy would you give Sandra?

5. Selene is five weeks pregnant and has developed morning sickness. She has dry heaves (2) and is irritable (3) in the morning with stomach cramps (2).
What is her remedy?

6. Sally is seven weeks pregnant and has morning sickness. She has retching (2) in the morning and feels better by eating (3). Her stomach always feels empty (1).
What is her remedy?

7. Teresa is one month pregnant and has developed severe morning sickness. She is vomiting all day (3) and has an aversion to food (2). Her nausea appears to be worse in a warm closed room (2).
What is her remedy?

READING ASSIGNMENT

Ipecacuanha / Ipecac. Materia Medica
Read Ipecac in the TEXT materia medica, p. 265 and on p. 76, in the chart on Nosebleed; also, if available, in your remedy kit brochure. Read Ipecac in BOERICKE on pp. 352 - 353, scanning the material by placing emphasis on finding the same symptoms in the TEXT. Read the modalities carefully.

WRITTEN ASSIGNMENT

Ipecacuanha / Ipecac. Materia Medica

8. How would you characterize the tongue and mouth in an Ipecac case of nausea and vomiting?

9. In an Ipecac nosebleed, what does the blood look like?

10. Write the abbreviation for Ipecac.

READING ASSIGNMENT

Read Varicose Veins p. 221 in the TEXT.

Note: If Hamamelis, used internally and externally, does not relieve the varicose veins, go to a homeopathic physician. A constitutional remedy may be able to relieve the condition. Surgery ought to be considered as the last resort.

Read pp. 221 - 222, Urinary Problems. Study each of the Cystitis remedies in the chart on pp. 230 - 240.

Cystitis Differential

Cantharis / Canth.
Cantharis is a commonly indicated acute cystitis remedy when there is frequent urination in small amounts and burning sensations during urination.

Pulsatilla / Puls.
The burning is not as intense as Cantharis. With Puls. the desire to urinate is increased when lying on the back in bed. Also there can be some involuntary dribbling of urine at night in bed from coughing, etc.

Staphysagria / Staph.
Is a physical trauma related cystitis remedy. Staphysagria is specific for 'honeymoon cystitis' resulting from sexual activity. There is a frequent urge to urinate. There are burning pains which are relieved during urination.

WRITTEN ASSIGNMENT

11. Sara is five months pregnant and has developed cystitis. She has to urinate often (2), but only a little comes out (3). She complains of burning pains (3) which are worse from urination (3).
What is her remedy? (Refer to BOERICKE for your answer.)

12. Which remedy comes to mind for cystitis arising from an etiology of excessive sexual activity, where the pains are relieved during urination?

READING ASSIGNMENT

Read pp. 222 - 224 in the TEXT up to Labor.

READING ASSIGNMENT

Coffea cruda / Coffea Materia Medica
Read Coffea in your remedy kit brochure, if available, and in BOERICKE on p. 222, scanning the material by placing emphasis on the introductory paragraph and the sections in Mind, Mouth, and Sleep, and the Modalities.

WRITTEN ASSIGNMENT

Coffea cruda / Coffea Materia Medica
13. What is the mood and energy state that would typify the Coffea insomnia?

14. What would temporarily relieve the Coffea toothache?

15. How do you imagine noise would affect the patient with a Coffea toothache?

16. Write the abbreviation for Coffea.

READING ASSIGNMENT

Read pp. 224 - 226 in the TEXT up to Breast Feeding.

Note: **Another remedy to consider for recovery from the trauma of childbirth is Bellis perennis. Bellis perennis is quite similar to Arnica; however Bellis is more specific for trauma to the pelvic organs. Think of Bellis for any trauma to the pelvic organs.**

READING ASSIGNMENT

Read pp. 226 - 227 in the TEXT, Breast Feeding. Read Phytolacca in the TEXT chart. Then study the supplemental material in the Syllabus which follows.

Nursing Guidelines

The nursing mother is advised to avoid or go easy on Brewers' yeast and B vitamins because they can give the child insomnia. If the mother is accustomed to taking herbal teas, she should then rotate at least four different kinds.

Alfalfa tincture may be applied to the breast as a tonic to prepare the breast for nursing. To prevent exhaustion from nursing and increase milk it is recommended that the mother take Lecithin and Alfalfa, as nutritional supplements.

Breast Feeding Differential

Aethusa cynapium / Aeth.
Milk is stringy. There is a bad taste and smell to the milk. Milk comes out in curds. The infant rejects the milk, or the milk is seemingly good but the child does not want it.

Agnus castus / Agn. / The Chaste Tree
Absence of sexual desire. There is scanty milk. The woman's face appears to be sad and shrivelled up. She is losing weight, has low energy and cold, clammy hands and feet.

Borax / Bor.
Has pains in the right breast when nursing on the left side. Severe aching when the breast is empty.

Rhus toxicodendron / Rhus. tox.
When baby starts nursing it is initially painful at first, but with continued nursing there is relief.

Calcarea carbonica / Calc.
Indicated for overnursing with loss of energy. Could have bad, scanty milk. The mother's metabolism is off. The breasts are achy, swollen, full, and heavy. Mother gains and loses weight easily.

Calcarea phosphorica / Calcarea phos. / Calc.-p.
Especially indicated where mother has poor nutrition. For women who smoke, drink coffee, and go back to work too soon. Breast and nipples are sore to touch. Milk is thin, watery, salty, and acrid. Children of the mother may develop weak bones or have severe teething problems.

Dulcamara / Dulc.
Milk stops, goes away after exposure to cold wet weather or feet getting wet. Mother could develop a sinus infection which goes to the breast and makes the whole apparatus of the breast inactive.

Kali bichromicum / Kali-bi.
Indicated for stringy, ropy, bad tasting milk.

Silicia / Sil.
Indicated for loss of energy due to overnursing. There is exhaustion, lack of stamina, and shortness of breath - this causes deficient milk. Silicia is more fragile than Calcarea.

Calendula Lotion
May be applied externally for cracked, tender, sore nipples.

Mastitis Differential
(Mastitis is inflammation of the breast)

Phytolacca / Phyt.
The main mastitis remedy. Hardness in breast. Nipples may be caked, cracked and sensitive. Breasts may feel better with support. Milk may be bloody or cheesy. There may be swollen glands in the neck.

Belladonna / Bell.
Indicated when there is high fever and much congestion, with redness in the breast. There could be red streaks in the breast from the nipple outward. Breasts are hot; they throb painfully and feel heavy.

Bryonia / Bry.
Breast is hard and heavy but pale. Sharp pain on moving the breast. The pain is better from pressure. Flow of milk is often diminished.

Hepar sulph / Hep.
Inflamed tender breast with sour smelling pus coming out.

Chamomilla / Cham.
Indicated for drawing pains, as if someone where pulling the breast or nipple off. Hard and tender breasts. Milk may be bloody or cheesy. Irritable, touchy and sleepless.

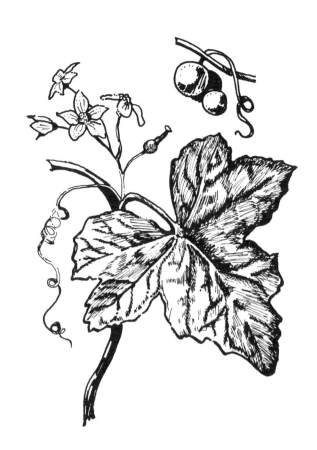

Bryonia alba

(Wild Hops)

WRITTEN ASSIGNMENT

17. The TEXT recommends Calcarea phos. for the stimulation of milk. What other natural supplements may be used to stimulate milk supply and prevent exhaustion?

18. Which remedy has stringy, ropy, bad tasting milk? Look this remedy up in BOERICKE to observe the similarity of the mucus discharges.

19. Which remedy finds beginning breast feeding initially painful but the discomfort is relieved from continued feeding? Find this remedy in Lesson 2 of the Syllabus to observe the same modalities.

READING ASSIGNMENT

Read Menopause, pp. 228 - 229 in the TEXT.

Dysmenorrhea or Painful Menstruation Differential

This following differential will be helpful in finding the acute remedy to relieve discomfort associated with menstruation. If the problem continues to recur, it is a sign of the need for deeper constitutional treatment by a homeopathic physician.

Magnesia phos. / Mag. phos.
Indicated for cramps and spasms which are better in heat and better from pressure. Mag phos. and Colocynthis are quite similar.

Colocynthis / Coloc.
Severe cramps. Sharp stabbing pains which are better from heat and pressing hard into the area. Wants to be left alone. Sensitive face distorted from pain. Pain comes and goes fast. Better bending forward - doubled up. Pain associated with anger.

Dioscorea / Dios. / Wild Yam
Better bending backwards, the opposite of Colocynthis. Cramps in the fingers and toes.

Belladonna / Bell.
Cramps, spasms, and bearing down pains come and go suddenly. There is heat and congestion. She is better sitting up and better from pressing of the genitals or abdomen. Worse from motion of any kind.

Borax / Bor.
Profuse early menses with griping pains and nausea. Pain in the stomach extends to the back. In the menstrual flow large membranes are passed. There may be nausea.

Cactus / Cact.
The whole uterus feels like a wire was wrapped around it and tightened, or as if squeezed by hand. The pains are constricting.

Caulophyllum / Caul.
Cramps in the uterus before menses, with pains in the lower back. There are bearing down spasmodic pains, with drawing pains in the legs. She feels weak and trembling inside. The uterus feels heavy and congested.

Cimicifuga racemosa / Cimicifuga / Cimic.
There are severe labor-like pains. Bearing down cramps and spasms. The pains travel from right to left to right, going back and forth. She bends over double and is restless, better from heat.

Sabina / Sabin.
Sharp pains travel from the sacrum (the back) to the pubic area (the front). The flow is red with clots. She desires fresh air and is warm blooded.

Lachesis / Lach.
Pains in the left ovary. There is sensitivity to any clothing where it binds at the neck or waist. The blackish menstrual flow relieves the symptoms.

Case Analysis Review

Let us review some aspects of case analysis covered in Lessons 4 and 5. In the actual experience of using homeopathy for an acute illness, one person could likely be displaying several acute complaints at the same time.

For example, a woman may have painful menstruation together with less intense symptoms of headache and nausea.

The best way to approach this situation is to identify the strongest symptom as an expression of the Chief Complaint, in this case the painful menses with its modalities.

Then we look to examine the possible Etiology, Onset, General, Mental / Emotional Symptoms and other specific Local Symptoms - headache and nausea. Our goal is to find one remedy which best matches *all* of the symptoms. However, we want to be sure the remedy we select will be indicated for the strongest symptom - the Chief Complaint - the painful menses.

What to Do with Chronic Symptoms if Encountered in Acute Prescribing

When using homeopathy for acutes, we take the present symptoms relating to the complaint and do not usually consider chronic symptoms.

For example: An adult with a case of Influenza whose symptoms correspond to Rhus tox. This person may also have been suffering from hemorrhoids for years. For the acute case we would not take the information of the chronic complaint with the acute symptoms. If the hemorrhoids have been around for a long time, it is a sign that they need to be considered part of a deep constitutional treatment from a homeopathic physician.

Since Lesson 5 we have covered much material on the various illnesses. It is suggested that you go back and review Case Analysis II in Lesson 5 before solving the following case.

WRITTEN ASSIGNMENT

20. Find the remedy for this case.
Rose, age 35.
My neighbor Rose describes her dysmenorrhea as a downward pressure (1) in the uterus. It is now noticed that she is almost going to cry, yet when she first entered the room was cheerful (3). She says the pain feels worse when lying down (2). When she walked across the street to mail a letter she felt some relief(1).
With the menstrual discomfort she is complaining of digestive troubles (3). Rose says the salad she had for lunch agreed well with her (2), but her dinner of vegetable stew did not (3). She says the stew does not feel like it is digesting well (3). There is a distension in her abdomen, with rumbling sounds (3).
Rose says she has a headache and it feels as if something were pressing on the top of her head (3).
Rose then goes on to display the eczema which she has had on her feet for the past five and a half years with crusty scabs that she says get worse in the winter.

READING ASSIGNMENT

Sulphur Materia Medica
Read Sulphur in the TEXT materia medica. Sulphur is a deep acting remedy usually prescribed by experienced homeopaths for chronic cases. Study of the role of Sulphur in chronic prescribing is beyond the scope of this course and should be reserved for more advanced courses. Sulphur is often indicated in dry, itching, burning skin conditions.

WRITTEN ASSIGNMENT

Sulphur Materia Medica
21. Why would a Sulphur uncover his feet in bed?

22. What are two characteristic sensations of Sulphur?

23. Does the Sulphur type like to bathe often?

24. How might a Sulphur skin condition smell?

READING ASSIGNMENT

Read pp. 241 - 245 in the TEXT.

Homeopathy for Pets

The use of homeopathy for animals is basically the same as for humans. When analyzing cases of animals we rely more upon our *observations* of the animal. Refer to the specific chapter in the TEXT which covers your pet's illness or complaint, and proceed with the case analysis as you normally would. If you intend to be using homeopathy for pets often, consider obtaining the recommended books for the treating of dogs and cats in Appendix B p. 130 Syllabus and on p. 281 TEXT.

How to Give a Remedy to an Animal

An ideal method is to obtain the remedy in lactose tablets, which dissolve instantly. A tiny spoon is the best way to give the remedy. A small spoonful, e.g. one half a teaspoon, may be placed on your pet's tongue. The remedy should be tapped out onto the spoon. You may use the cap, but care must be taken not to touch the remedy cap to the pet's mouth. If it is difficult to place the remedy on the pet's tongue, then you may attempt from the side to place it just between the lip and the gum. The animal will then dissolve it and lick it into the mouth.

If you only have the large pellets, one option would be to place the remedy inside a piece of bland bread and give that to the dog. In this case put more remedy, i.e. 10 large pellets size #35, into the bread to be sure the animal gets enough of the remedy. Remember, the idea is for the remedy to dissolve in the mouth.

Another way which works quite well is to dissolve the remedy in your pet's water, being sure it is chemical-free, so as to prevent antidoting of the remedy. The remedy could also be dissolved in milk.

Animals often respond dramatically to homeopathy. The TEXT gives samples of the scope of veterinary homeopathy. Here are two of my own:

Some friends have a very old tom cat who has been involved in fights all of his life. They moved to the country and brought this cat with them. Tom, the cat, was getting in fights with the neighbors' pack of young dogs. When I saw him he had lacerations on his head and face, was so sore and bruised that he could hardly walk. He looked like a flame about to go out. However, several doses of Arnica 30C given in his milk gave him a new lease on life within a week.

It was summertime and my neighbors' old dog was very hot and itching. She had managed to rub off the fur on her hind leg and some of the skin as well. The area was raw, red and oozing clear liquid. Infection appeared imminent. One dose of Sulphur dried up the area and put her on the road to recovery in half a day.

Perspective on the Bach Flower Remedies®

Many people who are interested in homeopathy ask about the Bach Flower Remedies®. Do they work? And what is their relation to homeopathy?

The Bach Flower Remedies® are derived mainly from trees and flowering plants. They are not prepared in exactly the same way as homeopathic remedies. Yet they do represent a subtle energetic medicine. Most Bach Remedies® are prepared by placing flowers in a clear glass bowl containing pure spring water, in the sun. Some of the energy from the flower is then imparted to the water and the remedy is made from this water and is preserved with alcohol.

There are 38 Bach Flower Remedies® and they are harmless and easy to use. Their sphere of action is mainly on the mental/emotional plane. They can be quite effective for alleviating negative moods and in temporarily balancing the personality. The action of these remedies is very delicate, and the negative mood tends to disappear unnoticed. Literature is available from the book dealers in Appendix D, which amply describes the moods for which the remedies are indicated. It is fairly simple to match the remedy to the mood. Bach Flower Remedies® come in liquid form and remedy kits are available from some homeopathic pharmacies.

Clinical experience tends to indicate that the Bach Flower Remedies® would not act as deeply as homeopathic remedies. If a Bach Flower Remedy® needs to be continually repeated for a given mood, which is only partially relieved, then it is a sign that a deep constitutional homeopathic treatment is needed to clear away the mood by its roots. The Bach Flower Remedies® can act beautifully, but compared to homeopathy their power is limited and short lived in most cases.

If you are under the care of a homeopath it is recommended that you refrain from experimenting with the Bach Flower Remedies® on yourself. It is advised that the Bach Flower Remedies® not be given at the same time with a homeopathic remedy. In this manner possible confusion is avoided; one can evaluate the results and know what the homeopathic remedy is doing.

COURSE CONCLUSION

It is hoped that this introductory course has served to whet your interest and that it will serve as an introduction to a deeper study of homeopathy. The Appendices which follow provide the needed resources.

Recommended Reading
A reading list of the most applicable works as an extension to this course is provided in Appendix A, p. 129. Additionally in the TEXT on pp. 280 - 283 there is a valuable recommended reading list.

Homeopathic Organizations and their Publications/Homeopathic Courses In-Person, are listed in Appendix B, p. 130. These resources offer a spectrum of informative services.

All the publications on the topic of Immunizations have been listed in Appendix C, p. 132.

Sources for Homeopathic Books
Listed in Appendix D, p. 134, are resources to provide practical access to the books you need.

Send to your instructor your responses to all of the written assignments from Lessons 11 and 12, together with any questions you may have.

Upon satisfactory completion of these last lessons, you will be sent the Homeopathic Medicine in the Home Certificate of Completion.

May you and your loved ones enjoy a high level of well-being through the help of homeopathy. May your knowledge and practical skills grow as you relieve suffering and help others achieve a high level of well-being with homeopathy.

May the vital force be with you!

APPENDIX A

RECOMMENDED READING

Acute Prescribing. By Robin Murphy, N.D., Seminar I. 8 tapes.
Presented in a practical format. Excellent for health professionals and serious lay homeopaths with some homeopathic experience. For ordering see Appendix D, p. 134.

Catching Good Health (With Homeopathic Medicine). By Raymond J. Garrett and TaRessa Stone.
New York: Carlton Press, Inc. 1987.
Of significant value for those interested in receiving homeopathic treatment for themselves or their family. This book is replete with moving personal accounts of homeopathic cures. The diseases cured include 'incurable cases,' chronic degenerative disease, physical pathology, and psychological imbalance.

Everybody's Guide to Homeopathic Medicines. By Stephen Cummings, F.N.P. and Dana Ullman, M.H.P. Los Angeles: Jeremy P. Tarcher, Inc., 1984.
This fine self-care book supplements the Course TEXT further specifying the point at which one should seek medical care, and also includes more medical information about the various acute illnesses.

Everyday Homeopathy. By Dr. David Gemmell. Beaconsfield, England:
Beaconsfield Publishers Ltd., 1987.
Recommended as a supplement to the Course TEXT. A new and excellent self-care book. Diagrams and remedy differentials for common ailments make the material highly accessible. Includes diagrams of when to seek medical assistance.

Homeopathy: Medicine of the New Man. By George Vithoulkas. New York:
Arco Publishing Inc., 1979.
An excellent introduction to homeopathy written by one of the greatest living homeopaths.

Kent's Repertory, Condensed Version edited by Julian Winston and Mitchell Shapiro, PA.
National Center for Homeopathy, 1990.
A simplified abbreviated form of Kent's Repertory useful for dealing with acute cases rapidly.

Practical Homeopathic Therapeutics. By W. A. Dewey, M.D. New Delhi, India:
B. Jain Reprint 1983.
A good supplementary book, full of valuable remedy differentials. The author was one of the eminent early American homeopathic medical doctors.

Science of Homeopathy, The. By George Vithoulkas. New York: Grove Press, 1980.
Indispensable for the serious intermediate and advanced student of homeopathy, this text offers a lucid exposition of homeopathic principles and philosophy along with practical applications.

Woman's Guide to Homeopathic Medicine, A. By Trevor Smith, M.D. New York:
Thorson's Publishers Inc., 1984.
A comprehensive book on homeopathy for women's complaints, of use for both beginning and advanced homeopaths.

Natural Health for Dogs and Cats. By Richard H. Pitcairn, D.V.M., PhD. and Susan Pitcairn, M.A.,
Emmaus, Pa: Rodale Press, 1982.
A thorough coverage of natural methods of prevention and health care with emphasis on homeopathy and nutrition.

The Homeopathic Treatment of Small Animals. By Christopher Day. London:
Wigmore Publications Limited, 1984.
One of the finest works on the subject to date. Useful for both veterinarians and pet owners.

APPENDIX B

HOMEOPATHIC ORGANIZATIONS - Their services and publications

HOMEOPATHIC COURSES - In-Person

Note - These two organizations listed first are marked with an asterisk (*). They have the most services and information to offer the beginner.

*International Foundation for Homeopathy (IFH)
2366 Eastlake Ave. E, Suite 301
Seattle, WA 98102
(206) 324-8230

A non-profit organization dedicated to promoting public awareness and researching the cost benefits of homeopathy, to maintain the highest standards of homeopathic practice and education; and towards the establishment of a homeopathic medical school. Membership includes subscription to Resonance, a bimonthly newsletter with informative articles and calendar of homeopathic educational opportunities. Offer a directory of competent licensed practitioners who use homeopathy consisting of those who have taken the IFH postgraduate training as well as other practitioners of good standards. Offers comprehensive postgraduate training in homeopathy for licensed health professionals as well as introductory courses to the public.

*National Center for Homeopathy (NCH)
1500 Massachusetts Avenue, N.W., Suite 41
Washington, D.C. 20005
(202) 223-6182

Serving as a central information center, this non-profit membership organization exists for the purpose of promoting homeopathy through education, publication, research and membership services. Membership includes an informative monthly publication, Homeopathy Today, which includes a national calendar of events and homeopathic educational opportunities. Offers a directory of licensed practitioners who use homeopathy. Offers a descriptive catalog of homeopathic books available to the public. Members receive discounts on purchases. The NCH provides annual summer courses in the following areas: courses for consumers on introductory, beginning, and intermediate levels; for licensed health care providers there is a dental course, veterinary course, chiropractic course, nurses' course, and an advanced professional course. Additionally, NCH offers periodical public seminars.

American Institute of Homeopathy
1500 Massachusetts Avenue, NW
Washington, DC 20005
(202) 223-6182

Affiliated with the National Center for Homeopathy, the American Institute of Homeopathy is the oldest national professional medical organization in the United States. Membership is open to licensed doctors of medicine, osteopathy and dentistry. The AIH has taken a leadership role in representing American Homeopathy before state and federal legislative and regulatory bodies. Membership includes the monthly AIH newsletter and the quarterly Journal of the American Institute of Homeopathy.

Foundation for Homeopathic Education and Research
5916 Chabot Crest
Oakland, CA 94618
(415) 649-8930

This non-profit foundation seeks funding to sponsor scientific research that will evaluate the biological and therapeutic action of homeopathic medicines. The Foundation disseminates results of these research projects within the scientific community and the general public. Its work includes interfacing with the media to accurately inform the general public about homeopathy. Homeopathic Research Reports, a newsletter of the Foundation provides an informative view of the Foundation's activities and goals.

Hahnemann College of Homeopathy
1918 Bonita Avenue
Berkeley, CA 94704
(415) 849-1925

Offers a two-year course which is the most advanced training in classical homeopathy that has been available in this country for over 50 years. The course is open to all licensed health practitioners and includes extensive training at the Hahnemann Medical Clinic.

HomeoNet
1386 San Anselmo Avenue
San Anselmo, CA 94960
(415) 457-0678

A computerized communications network of the world's homeopathic community. Of especial value to health practitioners and those having an intermediate understanding of homeopathy. Has an international calendar of homeopathic educational seminars and meetings. There is a bulletin board to provide homeopathic news, including that of study groups. The bookstore inexpensively offers a large selection of homeopathic books. The materia medica section offers original and historical articles on remedies with case quizzes. There is a journal of scholarly papers on research and homeopathic practice. A consulting bulletin board provides the forum to receive free advice on problem cases from other practitioners. There is a paid consulting service for consultation with some of the world's most respected homeopaths.

Homeopathic Academy of Naturopathic Physicians (HANP)
11231 S.E. Market St.
Portland, Oregon 97216

HANP exists to advance the scientific and clinical knowledge of homeopathy. It is also working to create and maintain continuing education for naturopathic physicians through board certification. Membership includes subscription to Similimum, a newsletter geared towards those having intermediate or advanced understanding of homeopathy.

National College of Naturopathic Medicine
11231 S.E. Market Street
Portland, Oregon 97216
(503) 255-4860

Their certification in homeopathy program is open to both students pursuing the N.D. degree and to certain qualified health professionals who wish to obtain a solid foundation in homeopathic prescribing.

Pacific Academy of Homeopathic Medicine
1678 Shattuck Ave. #42
Berkeley, CA 94709
(415) 549-3475

Founded to provide an opportunity for all student of homeopathy to learn from many diverse, excellent sources. Features periodic seminars with some of the world's finest teachers. The Essence, a newsletter of the academy, provides details of educational offerings.

APPENDIX C

RESOURCES ON IMMUNIZATIONS

American Natural Hygiene Society, The
12816 Race Track Road
Tampa, Florida 33625
(813) 855-6607
This organization provides yearly membership which offers school exemption letter formats which are applicable for children in all states. The publishing division of the society offers the following book:

> Allen, Hannah. *Don't Get Stuck! The Case Against Vaccinations and Injections.* National Hygiene Press, P.O. Box 1083, Oldsmar, Florida 33557. 1985.
> The book discusses how to legally avoid inoculations and protect your rights. It provides information on immunity and vaccinal antibodies.

Coulter, Harris L., and Fisher, Barbara Loe. *DPT: A Shot in the Dark.* San Diego, New York, London: Harcourt Brace Jovanovich, 1985.
An exposé of the harmful effects of the DPT vaccine. Includes moving personal accounts relating to vaccine-injured children and studies the value and safety of the pertussis vaccine.

Dissatisfied Parents Together (DPT)
128 Branch Road
Vienna, VA 22180
(703) 983- DPT3
This organization exists to provide information to help parents make informed decisions about vaccines. Offers yearly membership with newsletter.

Finn, Tom, Attorney. *Dangers of Compulsory Immunizations - How To Avoid Them Legally.* Family Fitness Press, P.O. Box 1658, New Port Richey, Florida 33552, 1983. (813) 376-1208
An informative and well written book covers the legal issue of avoiding immunizations with astute clarity.

Girdwain, Grace. How to Legally Avoid Immunizations of All Kinds.
Humanitarian Publishing Company, R.D. #3, Clymer Road, Quakertown, PA 18951.
(215) 536-1900.
This booklet informs the reader of the legal rights to refuse vaccinations and explains how to exercise those rights.

James, Walene. *Immunization: The Reality Behind the Myth.*
Bergin & Garvey, 1988.
Exposes the existing medical model and offers the perspective of a new model of reality relating to vaccinations.

Mothering Magazine. Immunizations - A Mothering Publication's Special Edition.
Mothering Magazine, P.O. Box 8410, Sante Fe, New Mexico 87504.
A comprehensive and informative compilation of articles on the subject of immunizations. Recommended.

National Center for Homeopathy
1500 Massachusetts Ave., NW
Washington, DC 20005
(202) 223-6182
A central information center. They offer yearly membership with newsletter and provides the following relevant booklets:

Nossaman, Nicholas, M.D. <u>More About Immunizations.</u>

Practical booklet discusses the immunizations given in childhood with a balanced presentation on clinical diseases, their statistics, the current vaccines and possible side effects.

Moskowitz, Richard, M.D., D.Ht. <u>The Case Against Immunizations.</u>

This booklet provides statistical information relating to the decline of childhood diseases in relation to the introduction of immunizations. Includes case histories demonstrating the side effects and medical complications associated with vaccination.

National Health Federation, The
212 W. Foothill Blvd.
P.O. Box 688
Monrovia, CA 91016
(818) 357-2181
Offers an immunization information kit which provides information on immunizations, their dangers, how to avoid them, and certificate of exemption.

Neustaedter, Randall, O.M.D., C.A. *The Immunization Decision: A Guide for Parents*
North Atlantic Books, 2320 Blake St., Berkeley, CA 94704
The most informative book on vaccines available to date. It comprehensively covers each disease, the efficacy of corresponding vaccines, side effects, and recommendations. Provides the reader with a basis for decision making on this issue. Recommended.

Vithoulkas, George. *The Science of Homeopathy*. New York: Grove Press, Inc., 1980.
This comprehensive text offers a scientific and in-depth analysis of the possibilities which can occur within the health of an individual as a result of vaccination.

For ordering these books - where not otherwise indicated, see Appendix D for sources which supply homeopathic books.

APPENDIX D

SOURCES FOR HOMEOPATHIC BOOKS

Boiron/Borneman
1208 Amosland Rd.
Norwood, PA 19074
(215) 532-2035 (inside PA.)
1-800 BLU-TUBE (Out-of-State)

B. Jain Publishers
1921, 10th St., Chuna Mandi
Pahar Ganj, New Delhi 110055
India

Center for the Distribution of Classical Homeopathic Literature
J. van Twillert
Da Costalaan 20, 3852 BN Ermelo
The Netherlands

Dolisos
3014 Rigel Ave.
Las Vegas, Nevada 89103
(702) 871-7153 (inside Nevada)
1-800-824-8455 (Out-of-State)

Ehrhart and Karl, Inc.
33 N. Wabash Avenue, Suite 316
Chicago, IL 60602
(312) 332-1046

Homeopathic Educational Services
2036 Blake St.
Berkeley, CA 94704
(415) 649-0294

Luyties Pharmacal Company
4200 Laclede Ave.
St. Louis, Missouri 63108
(314) 652-8080 (inside Missouri)
1-800-325-8080 (Out-of-State)

Robin Murphy, N.D.
2801 Rodeo Rd., Suite B-135
Santa Fe, New Mexico 87505
(505) 989-7018
Taped lecture Series.

National Center for Homeopathy
1500 Massachusetts Avenue, N.W., Suite 41
Washington, DC 20005
(202) 223-6182

Standard Homeopathic Company
Book Department
P.O. Box 61067
Los Angeles, CA 90061
1-800-624-9659

APPENDIX E

GUIDELINES FOR THE LOCATION AND SELECTION OF A HOMEOPATHIC PHYSICIAN/PRACTITIONER

Although there is no one guaranteed foolproof formula for selecting a competent homeopathic physician/practitioner, it is hoped that these guidelines will help in the selection process.

How to Locate Homeopaths in your Area

The International Foundation of Homeopathy, 2366 Eastlake Ave. E, Suite 301, Seattle, WA 98102, (206) 324-8230, publishes a directory of competent licensed practitioners consisting of those who have taken the IFH postgraduate training as well as other practitioners of good standards. Contact the IFH for information.

The National Center for Homeopathy, 1500 Massachusetts Ave., NW, Washington, D.C. 20005, (202) 223-6182, publishes an inexpensive directory of licensed practitioners who use homeopathy. However, this directory does not provide evaluation of the competency of practitioners listed therein.

If you cannot find a homeopath listed in your vicinity, repair with the directories to an atlas of the U.S. Often you will be able to find someone in a neighboring city or state who is within driving distance.
Ask the managment of health food stores, herb stores, holistic book-stores and centers, etc., in your area. They will often know of the presence of homeopaths.
Check in local or regional holistic health oriented papers and magazines. Some of them have directories which list practitioners. Homeopaths can often be found listed there.

Guidelines for Deciding Who is the Most Competent

* When using the National Center of Homeopathy Directory of Homeopathic Practitioners there is a code which indicates to what percentage each practitioner uses homeopathy. Favor selection of those practitioners who practice homeopathy predominantly. Naturally those practitioners who use homeopathy more often will tend to be more experienced.

* Check to see where and with whom the homeopath trained. If the training was in the United States, check to see if it was with trainings listed in Appendix B of the Syllabus. Those are among the best trainings in the U.S. Find out how long the practitioner has studied homeopathy, if he or she had an internship and how long he or she has been practicing.

* In making your selection favor the homeopath who gives one remedy at a time, taking great consideration and care to evaluate the totality of symptoms on all levels - mentally, emotionally and physically.

* In making your selection avoid the physician or practitioner who as a rule gives many homeopathic remedies at a time and/or who always mixes homeopathy with numerous other healing modalities such as herbs and therapeutic doses of vitamins. A competent homeopath will as a rule be able to effect deep long lasting results giving one remedy at a time.

* Feedback and word-of-mouth from others in your area can also be helpful in your selection process.

In some cases it may not be possible to locate a competent homeopathic physician/practitioner in your immediate vicinity. In this situation it is worthwhile to make the commitment to travel to a practitioner who is qualified and competent who will be able to help deeply.

REFERENCES

Allen, H.C. *Allen's Keynotes & Characteristics of the Materia Medica with Nosodes.*
New Delhi: Jain Publishing Co., 1980.

Berkow, Robert. *The Merck Manual.*
Rahway: Merck Sharp & Dohme Research Laboratories, 1977.

Boericke, William. *Materia Medica with Repertory.*
New Delhi: Jain Publishing Co., 1980.

Borland, Douglas M. *Children's Types.*
New Delhi: World Homeopathic Links.

Clarke, John Henry. *A Dictionary of Practical Materia Medica.*
New Delhi: Jain Publishing Co., 1978.

Coulter, Harris L. *The Physics of Healing with Microdoses.*
Berkeley: North Atlantic Books, 1980.

Coulter, Harris L., and Fisher, Barbara Loe. *DPT: A Shot in the Dark.*
San Diego, New York, London: Harcourt Brace Jovanovich, 1985.

Cummings, Steven, and Ullman, Dana. *Everybody's Guide to Homeopathic Medicines.*
Los Angeles: Jeremy P. Tarcher, Inc., 1984.

Dewey, W.A. *Practical Homeopathic Therapeutics.*
New Delhi: Jain Publishing Co., 1983

Dhawale, M.L. *Principles and Practice of Homeopathy.*
Bombay: Institute of Clinical Research, 1985.

Girdwain, Grace. *How to Legally Avoid Immunizations of All Kinds.*
Quakertown, PA: Humanitarian Publishing Company,

Grassi, Maggi Lidchi. *The Spiritual Implications of Homeopathic Medicine.*
McAfee, New Jersey: Assembly of the World's Religions, 1985.

Kent, James Tyler. *Lectures on Homeopathic Materia Medica.*
New Delhi: Jain Publishing Co., 1982

Kent, James Tyler. *Repertory of the Homeopathic Materia Medica.*
Calcutta: Sett Dey & Co., 1961

Macleod, George. *The Homeopathic Treatment of Dogs.*
London: The Homeopathic Development Foundation Ltd., 1983.

Montessori, Maria. *The Absorbent Mind.*
Madras: Kalakshetra Publications, 1973.

Murphy, Robin. *The Fundamentals of Classical Homeopathy - Lecture Series.*
References specifically drawn from Acute Prescribing I, II, and III, Pediatrics, Women's Health Care, Homeopathy for Psychological Problems, Treatment of Dermatological Disorders, and Gastroenterology.

Neustaedter, Randy *et al. Immunizations: Are They Necessary?*
Hering Family Health Clinic, 1981.

Ortega, Proceso S. *Notes on the Miasms.*
New Delhi: National Homeopathic Pharmacy, 1983.

Roberts, Herbert A. *The Principles and Art of Cure by Homeopathy.*
Devon, England, 1942.

Stuller, Jay. *Duck/Flu Season, Quack...Quack...Quack-choo!*
American Health Magazine, December 1987, p.8.

Taber, Clarence Wilbur. *Taber's Cyclopedic Medical Dictionary.*
Philadelphia: F.A. Davis Company, 1981.

Tyler, Margaret L., M.D. *Homeopathic Drug Pictures.*

Devon, England: Health Science Press, 1952.

Vithoulkas, George. *Homeopathy: Medicine of the New Man.*
New York: Arco Publishing, 1979.

Vithoulkas, George. *The Science of Homeopathy.*
New York: Grove Press, Inc., 1980

Weeks, Nora. *The Medical Discoveries of Edward Bach, Physician - What the Flowers do for the Human Body* London: The C.W. Daniel Company Ltd., 1952.

Whitmont, Edward C. *Psyche & Substance: Essays on Homeopathy in the Light of Jungian Psychology.*
Richmond, California: North Atlantic Books, 1980.

Wright-Hubbard Elizabeth. *A Brief Study Course in Homeopathy.*
St. Louis: Formur Inc., 1977.

GLOSSARY

Acute Illness
A complaint of temporary duration of usually less than three weeks time which can be treated at home using self-care.

C Potency
A homeopathic remedy which has been diluted on the centesimal scale, which is one part of original substance to 99 parts diluting medium.

Chief Complaint
The general name of the main or predominant illness in a case, which is usually ascertained during casetaking and listed first in the format for recorded symptoms.

Chronic Illness
An illness which has been in existence for more than one month and is an expression of a deep seated ongoing imbalance. Chronic illnesses require a deep constitutional homeopathic treatment and should be handled by a homeopathic physician.

Colic
A spasmodic pain in any soft organ. In infants this pain is commonly seen in the abdomen and is related to a digestive upset.

Constitutional homeopathic treatment
A form of homeopathic treatment prescribed by a competent homeopathic physician which takes into consideration the totality of a person's symptoms and attributes on the mental, emotional, and physical levels. The constitutional homeopathic remedy is given to effect a deep balancing in the energetic metabolism of a person. The effects of such treatment can continue to work for months and even years, acting deeply on resolving long standing imbalances of health in accordance with Hering's laws of cure.

Cyanosis
A bluish, grayish, or purple discoloration in the skin caused by a deficiency of oxygen. Relating to childbirth, it refers to new-born infants whose skin is cyanotic; who are not getting enough oxygen.

Cystitis
Inflammation of the bladder. Frequent and painful urination is often present.

Dysmenorrhea
Painful or difficult menstruation. Symptoms of pain in the uterus or ovaries, abdominal distention, headaches, nausea, soreness of breasts, back or legs - may be present just prior to the onset of or during menstruation.

Enuresis
Involuntary urination. This is most commonly seen in children as bedwetting.

General Symptoms
Those symptoms which are an expression of the 'overall' general body characteristics. The most common general symptoms seen in minor ailments include body temperature reactions, the energy level, appearance of the skin, degree of thirst, food cravings or aversions, and perspiration.

Hering's Laws of Cure
Natural laws of healing which state that healing occurs at the deepest levels first and proceeds through to less serious levels on the periphery of the physical plane. On the physical plane cure proceeds going from the nervous system and vital organs toward the skin. And on the skin going from the head toward the feet. Previously experienced ailments reappear and then disappear, from the most recent going back in time chronologically.

Hierachy of Health
The schema for understanding the relative depth of illness in the three interrelated planes of health - mental, emotional and physical. The general concept is that the mental plane represents the deepest level of health while the emotional plane is the next in depth and the physical plane, although important, is more on the periphery of the organism.

Law of Similars
The vital principle upon which homeopathy is based; similia similibus curentur - like cures like. By giving to a sick person that substance which can cause the same symptoms in a healthy person, a curative natural healing response takes place.

Local Symptoms
Detailed characteristics in a case which relate to the particular manifestations of illness. The main local symptoms are these: Location of symptoms, sensations, discharges, and modalities.

Lotion
A mild liquid preparation, usually for external application, which is made by diluting a liquid vegetal tincture, (i.e. one part tincture to four parts water), to take the sting out of the tincture due to its high alcohol content.

Malabsorption syndrome
A disordered absorption of nutrients in the intestinal tract. Relating to infancy, this is commonly seen as an intolerance for mother's milk and milk in general, which can cause diarrhea and vomiting.

Mastitis
Inflammation of the breast. Most commonly seen in women during breast feeding or lactation.

Materia Medica
The detailed characteristics, unique properties, and indications for use of each homeopathic medicine. Reference books which house this information are known as *materia medicas*.

Mental/Emotional State
The outstanding psychological attributes of a person. In acute casetaking one looks for these outstanding psychological traits which are unique to the time of the acute illness.

Modalities
Any conditions which make the symptoms better or worse.

Morning Sickness
Symptoms of nausea and vomiting which occur during the first few months of pregnancy, expecially in the moring.

Multiple Symptom Case
An illness where the Chief Complaint has more than one area of symptomatology. For example, Influenza having headache, sore throat and congestion in chest.

Onset
The characteristic manner in which an illness develops, i.e. slow or rapid.

Personality Picture
Homeopathic materia medica which focuses on the mental/emotional attributes of a homeopathic remedy showing its relationship to the psychological state of man or beast.

Plussing
A technique of increasing the potency of a homeopathic remedy. The remedy is dissolved in water, and through a process of repeated dilution and stirring of the solution the potency is increased.

Polychrest
A homeopathic remedy with a wide range of applicability that makes it readily usable.

Potentization
The process through which a homeopathic remedy is manufactured. Through repeated dilution of the original substance coupled with succusssion (shaking of the dilution), the original substance is transformed into a dynamized energetic representation of the original substance.

Repertory
A homeopathic reference work which, in great detail, lists all known symptoms and attributes, with abbreviations of the remedies that correspond to them.

Similimum
That homeopathic remedy which most completely matches the totality of an individual's symptoms and attributes.

Succussion
A vital part of the process of potentization in the making of a homeopathic remedy. During succussion the diluted solution is vigorously shaken by striking a firm surface.

Suppression
A process whereby the state of health of an individual is manipulated by various therapy(ies) which drive the symptoms of illness into deeper levels, in a direction opposite to Hering's laws of cure. The result is that the immediate set of symptoms disappear and the individual then becomes more unhealthy and disposed to develop more serious manifestations of illness on deeper levels.

Tincture
A liquid vegetal extract in an alcohol solution.

Vesicular eruption
Eruptions of small blisters on the skin, commonly seen in herpes and poison ivy or oak eruptions.

Vital Force
The underlying energy which represents the core of an individual's health. In western medicine the closest synonym is the immunological defense mechanism and in oriental medicine, chi.

X Potency
A homeopathy remedy which has been diluted in the decimal scale which is one part of original substance to nine parts diluting medium.

INDEX